**BRADY**

# EMERGENCY FIRST CARE

## FIRST AID AND CPR GUIDE FOR WORKERS, FAMILIES, AND BYSTANDERS

## Frank J. Poliafico, R.N.

D1383588

**BRADY**
**Prentice Hall**
Upper Saddle River, New Jersey 07458

*Library of Congress Cataloging-in-Publication Data*
Poliafico, Frank J.
    Emergency first care: first aid and CPR guide for workers,
    families, and bystanders/Frank J. Poliafico.
        p.    cm.
    ISBN 0-89303-181-X (p)
    1. First aid in illness and injury.    2. CPR (First aid)
    I. Title
    RC86.7.P65    1996
616.02'52—dc20                                    95–42712

Publisher: *Susan Katz*
Editorial Assistant: *Carol Sobel*
Marketing Manager: *Judy Streger*
Director of Production and Manufacturing: *Bruce Johnson*
Managing Production Editor: *Patrick Walsh*
Production Editor: *Julie Boddorf*
Production Coordinators: *Ed O'Dougherty/Ilene Sanford*
Cover Designer: *Laura Ierardi*
Cover Photography: *The Stock Market/Lightscapes*
Managing Photography Editor: *Michal Heron*
Photographer: *Michael O'Neill*
Printer/Binder: *The Banta Company, Menasha, Wisconsin*

 © 1996 by Frank J. Poliafico

Printed in the United States of America

10   9   8   7   6   5   4   3   2   1

ISBN 0-89303-181-X

PRENTICE-HALL INTERNATIONAL (UK) LIMITED, *London*
PRENTICE-HALL OF AUSTRALIA PTY. LIMITED, *Sydney*
PRENTICE-HALL CANADA INC., *Toronto*
PRENTICE HALL HISPANOAMERICANA, S.A., *Mexico*
PRENTICE-HALL OF INDIA PRIVATE LIMITED, *New Delhi*
PRENTICE-HALL OF JAPAN, INC., *Tokyo*
SIMON & SCHUSTER ASIA PTE. LTD., *Singapore*
EDITORA PRENTICE-HALL DO BRASIL, LTDA., *Rio de Janeiro*

Dedicated to the nurses who taught me to care:

Dorothy Stewart Thompson, R.N.
Eleanor Dower, R.N.
Katherine Melwert, R.N.
Ann Agner, R.N.*
Margaret Simoncelli, R.N.*

and the one who showed me how to teach:

James P. Healy, R.N.*

and to my friend and mentor who inspired me to write:

Harvey D. Grant*

*May they rest in peace.

# CONTENTS

# PART 3

## CARE UNTIL PROFESSIONAL MEDICAL HELP IS AVAILABLE   77

# PART 4

## LIFE SUPPORT FOR SUDDEN DEATH   95

# PART 5

## PUTTING IT ALL TOGETHER   121

# FOREWORD

About one-fourth of all deaths in developed industrialized countries during peace time occur acutely, before one's time has come. Such deaths are a result of sudden critical injury or illness, without underlying incurable disease, and before the onset of old age or severe senility. A large proportion of these deaths and many additional cases of accidental crippling could be avoided by maximal application of modern resuscitation and life support. The role of the lay person is critical.

Before the 1950s, there were no effective methods for use by non-medical persons to reverse upper air-passage obstruction in coma (which invariably occurs when the head is not held tilted backward), cessation of breathing, or cessation of heart beat (pulselessness). Since that time, through the efforts of several physicians and scientists, the cardiopulmonary-cerebral resuscitation (CPCR) system was developed. The system consists of basic, advanced, and prolonged life support (BLS-ALS-PLS). It is applied through a "life support chain," individual life support actions by persons acting together as a linked "chain of survival." The links begin at the scene of the emergency with life support provided by a bystander, who as soon as feasible calls the 911 operator, who sends the ambulance crew, who provide ongoing life support and transport to the most appropriate hospital. Any chain is only as good as its weakest link.

Unfortunately, the weakest link in the "chain of survival" has been care by bystanders. It is family, friends, co-workers, and passers-by who are usually the first to determine the need for immediate "life-supporting first aid" (LSFA) at the scene of a medical or surgical emergency, and the ones who must provide it. LSFA consists of approximately eight simple steps (as shown in the figure on page xi). These include cardiopulmonary resuscitation (CPR) steps A (airway control), B (mouth-to-mouth breathing), and C (circulation support by chest compressions); control of severe external bleeding; positioning the person for shock and coma; and calling for help.

I suspect that steps A and B alone, for comatose victims with a pulse, have saved more lives than chest compressions for pulselessness. When in doubt, start life support and continue until a health professional takes over. The "AIDS paranoia" should not prevent mouth-to-mouth breathing. I encourage you to carry in your pocket a simple barrier for resuscitating strangers. When resuscitating previously healthy relatives or friends, do not worry about infection.

Simplicity in teaching is critical to remember the essentials of LSFA: "If unconscious, tilt head back. If no breathing, breathe mouth-to-mouth. If no pulse, circulate by pushing on the breast bone. If external bleeding, compress and elevate. If in coma or shock, place victim horizontal with legs up and head tilted back" (we have promoted these simple instructions since the 1960s!). Even partial acquisition of these skills by millions of people would save more lives than "military drill" practice to perfection by few.

The life saving potential of LSFA is evident; however, there is still a large gap between what is known about saving lives and what is applied in actual practice in the community everyday. In communities where bystander CPR is given for sudden death, survival rates are significantly higher than in communities where CPR attempts are delayed until the ambulance team arrives. Some trauma victims still bleed to death from external hemorrhage. Some head trauma victims with potentially non-crippling initial brain injury still end up permanently incapacitated because transient loss of airway and breathing at the scene were not controlled by bystanders with backward tilt of the head and mouth-to-mouth (or in case of tight jaw, mouth-to-nose) breathing.

Based on education research, some of us have promoted since the 1960s widespread training in LSFA from school age to old age. We also believe that such training should be a requirement for licensing drivers. In spite of many good courses available with lectures, slide shows, and instructor-coached manikin practice to perfection, such broadly based public capability has not yet been achieved. Moreover, such courses are expensive and have reached few.

Although programs can be useful, LSFA skills *can* be acquired through simpler, inexpensive self-training. This might include motivating television spots, repetitive viewing of demonstration films or videos, and self-practice (in families or small groups) of some steps on inexpensive manikins and other steps on one another, all coached by audiotape or videotape.

CPR guidelines on "what to teach" non-medical persons were formulated in the 1960s by the National Research Council (NRC) and since the 1970s by the American Heart Association (AHA). The American Red Cross (ARC) and its chapters adopted the AHA CPR guidelines and added many other first aid measures. Such guidelines for lay persons should be uniform and ideally be based on scientific evidence. Where scientific evidence is lacking, minor differences are unavoidable, such as between this book, *Emergency First Care*, the manuals of the ARC and AHA, and my own views.

With respect to "whom to teach" and "how to teach," uniformity is not required, and I encourage diversification and experimentation. In spite of laudable efforts with guidelines and formal courses, national organizations which have assumed responsibility for public education in first aid and CPR over the past 30 years, have not achieved the desired near 100% response rate by bystanders witnessing life threatening emergencies outside hospitals. In the United States, even in some resuscitation conscious communities, only about one-third of sudden deaths receive bystander CPR. The ARC and AHA need help.

This book, *Emergency First Care*, by Frank J. Poliafico, an experienced emergency nurse and educator, should not be viewed as competing with ARC manuals, but rather as complementing them. This book also deals with some non-life threatening medical emergencies, as do ARC and other manuals. The author also promotes prevention, which is laudable. I did not review and critique the details of this book. Readers of this book should realize that being prepared to help save a life through LSFA is far more important than learning how to bandage minor wounds or splint limb injuries. Moreover, LSFA can be applied without book or manual in hand.

What about the future? Researchers are now creating exciting possibilities for "saving hearts and brains too good to die" (C. Beck, P. Safar). In sudden deaths, many hearts are too sick to respond to attempts at restarting them in the field; and many brains are doomed because of late CPR. Permanent brain damage occurs after as little as 4 minutes of heart arrest. In the 21st century, "what" LSFA actions (skills) to teach lay persons may be modified. Future changes may include: mild cooling of the head or whole body to preserve brain viability in unconscious victims; automatic external defibrillation of heart arrest victims by non-medical persons; use of tourniquet for severe bleeding from extremities; and perhaps even medications by first responders. All this is still experimental. The key challenge for bystanders remains keeping the heart and brain alive with vigorous, immediately initiated steps A-B-C, until paramedics or physicians arrive with their increasingly sophisticated "tricks" to save lives.

What bystanders can do in emergencies is extremely important. The quicker and better you initiate emergency resuscitation, the less the victim will need expensive, prolonged (often futile), in-hospital intensive care. Whenever you try to participate in saving another life, you enhance the meaning of your own life. If you fail in your attempts, do not despair. Often the insult is beyond repair or the emergency occurred unwitnessed and help came too late. Whatever the outcome, your attempt to save a life means a triumph of the human spirit over the often cruel random chances of nature.

*Peter Safar, M.D., Dr.h.c., F.C.C.M., F.C.C.P.*
*SCRR, University of Pittsburgh*

# LIFE SUPPORTING FIRST AID
## (keep this card near areas of possible need)

**1**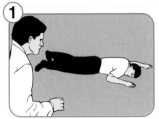

### SURVEY THE SCENE:
- Be certain it is safe to approach
  If not safe, call an ambulance
- Do not move a victim unless absolutely necessary

**2**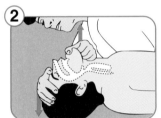

### IF UNCONSCIOUS:
- Tilt head back gently
- Lift chin, open mouth
- Look for chest movement, listen and feel for a flow from mouth/nose

**3**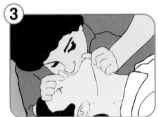

### IF NOT BREATHING:
- Pinch nose
- Make mouth to mouth seal
- Breathe slowly until victim's chest rises
- Give one breath every 5 seconds

**4**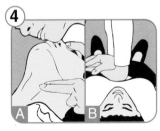

### IF NO PULSE:
- Place heels of hands, one on top of the other, just below the center of the breastbone
- Compress the chest about 15 times in about 10 seconds
- Alternate 2 breaths and 15 compressions until ambulance crew arrives

**5**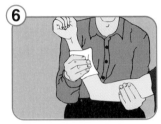

### IF CHOKING:
- Place fist just above navel
- Thrust inward and upward
- Repeat until object is dislodged

**6**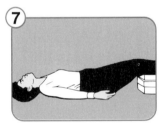

### IF BLEEDING:
- Apply pressure over the wound
- Place a gauze pad or cloth over the wound if available
- Elevate the wound if it does not cause pain
- Bandage the wound

**7**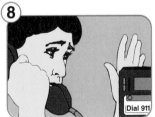

### MINIMIZE SHOCK:
- Place victim on back
- Keep head straight
- Elevate legs
- If unconscious, hold head tilted back

**8**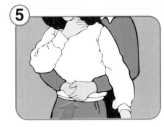

### CALL AN AMBULANCE:
- Send someone to call 9-1-1 or other local emergency number _____
- Tell the dispatcher the following:
  - Your name
  - Location of emergency
  - Type of emergency
  - Phone number calling from
- Stay on the line for instructions

---

## Call Emergency Medical Services (EMS) should any of these emergencies arise:
• Drowning • Electrical shock • Choking • Chest or abdominal pain • Severe pain • Severe/prolonged headache and/or diminished consciousness • Poisoning • Falls or impact • Severe bleeding • Unconsciousness • Difficulty or no breathing • Weak or no pulse • Major injury

Safar Center for Resuscitation Research
University of Pittsburgh

# PREFACE

The best way to deal with a medical emergency is to prevent it! Nevertheless, a serious illness or injury can happen anywhere, at any time, to anyone. In 1971 the Brady Publishing Company released the first edition of *Emergency Care*. This text became a cornerstone of Emergency Medical Technician (EMT) training and more than 20 years of dramatic prehospital emergency medical care advances. With the publication of *Emergency First Care* it is our goal to reinforce the foundation of effective Emergency Medical Systems.

Properly trained emergency medical professionals are rarely the ones who first encounter and attend to a sick or injured person's medical needs. Despite numerous improvements in the field of EMS, the outcome of medical emergencies is often determined not only by EMTs, paramedics, emergency nurses, or trauma surgeons but also by family members, coworkers, and other individuals who usually are the first people to detect and respond to a medical emergency.

When a sudden illness or injury occurs, modern paramedic ambulances and medical centers can be 10 to 30 minutes distant, if not more. Whether or not sophisticated medical services are available on-site when a medical emergency occurs, the application of simple assessment and life support procedures by trained and properly directed nonmedical personnel until professional help is available has proved effective in controlling the physical and fiscal complications of a serious illness or injury, as well as assuring the likelihood of a person's survival.

Emergency medical experts acknowledge that the weakest link in community EMS systems is public education: how to properly access the system and what to do until a land or air ambulance arrives. The idea of nonmedical people giving immediate aid to the victim of an accident or sudden illness is not new. However, programs designed to prepare lay responders for medical emergencies are often antiquated, inadequate, not relevant to a particular work setting, and/or not readily available

Leading emergency medical education experts have noted that traditional emergency care programs for nonclinicians have not been very effective for two primary reasons: these programs tend to be too technical, often teaching the wrong things, and teaching methods are poorly matched to the needs of average citizens. In an address before the Emergency Cardiac Care Update Conference in May of 1994, Dr. Peter Safer, the "Father of Modern Day Resuscitation," restated the need for, and the importance of, simplified first aid and CPR training. He called for a unified Life Support First Aid (LSFA) program "for hearts and brains too good to die." An uncomplicated, effective, and convenient emergency care training program is especially needed in industrial and occupational settings.

*Emergency First Care* was created to help meet this glaring deficiency in the workplace and elsewhere. *Emergency First Care* is designed to help nonmedical people develop skills and confidence to support life in persons who are perceived to have suffered a serious medical event (illness or trauma) until professional medical care is available. *Emergency First Care* is an up-to-date, practical, and effective answer to the need for an educationally sound and medically appropriate emergency training program for anyone who is likely to arrive first at the side of a sick or injured person.

*Emergency First Care* teaches life support for the clinically dead (CPR) according to the guidelines of the National Conference on Standards for Cardiopulmonary Resuscitation and Emergency Cardiac Care as published in the Journal of the American Medical Association. More importantly, it applies the same general principles of life support to help the "not yet dead." In *Emergency First Care*, the ABC'S plan is expanded to support life in someone who is physiologically compromised but has not deteriorated to the point of sudden death. By maintaining a person's open and clear **A**irway, assisting the process of **B**reathing, supporting the functions of **C**irculation, and supporting the structure of the **Spine**, a First Care giver can simply and safely provide effective assistance in the event of a perceived medical emergency and can very possibly prevent sudden death from occurring.

*Emergency First Care* meets or exceeds standards and requirements for the emergency care training of nonmedical workers set by OSHA, the FAA, the U.S. Coast Guard, and other agencies. It closely adheres to the Department of Transportation guidelines for "bystander care." It can also fulfill "right-to-know" and "blood-borne pathogen" legislated requirements for instructing employees in emergency medical care procedures.

Since 1979, this internationally acclaimed program has been utilized by numerous major companies on land, at sea, and in the sky. The content and approach follow proven, educationally sound principles for maximum participant motivation, learning, and skills retention.

## ABOUT THIS BOOK

This action guide is created to help you learn, reinforce, and practice the behaviors of immediate care for someone seriously ill or injured. It is primarily intended as a supplement to basic emergency medical training such as an Emergency First Care program conducted by experienced and qualified instructors. It will also serve as an ideal review and quick reference for individuals trained in all first aid and CPR programs.

It should be noted that information and procedures described are based on current, generally accepted principles of emergency medical care. However, application may vary as unusual circumstances or hazardous conditions arise. Neither this material nor other information provided in an Emergency First Care program is intended as a substitute for professional medical care.

In this book there are 16 chapters. The core material is presented in four major topical sections:

1. *Patient Care Actions*
   The primary text, illustrations, and graphics of *Emergency First Care* are designed to give you a reasonable and appropriate plan of action at the time of a perceived emergency.

2. *Helpful Background Information*
   *Emergency First Care* is primarily focused on what you *do*, not what you *know*. Nevertheless, these tinted areas will give you basic information and rationale for the actions indicated.

3. *Myths and Misconceptions*

   The history of first aid and CPR contains many old wives' tales and home remedies. Most of these are at best ineffective and at worst inappropriate or dangerous. Some are based on half-truths; others are "just the way we've always done it."

   Modern-day emergency medicine and the advances of such medical specialties as cardiac, burn, and trauma care have dispelled some of these old myths and, in other cases, have introduced a better way.

   In the shaded areas of each unit we will briefly discuss the most common misconceptions and why they are inappropriate or no longer relevant.

4. *Don't Let It Happen to You!*

   Most serious illnesses and all accidents are preventable! Throughout this book we will focus on being ready for these situations. We will also offer you suggestions and medically accepted principles to help you be healthy and safe.

   No portion of this document may be reproduced or reprinted without the express written permission of Frank J. Poliafico, R.N.

*Frank J. Poliafico, R.N.*
*Emergency & Safety Programs, Inc.*
*00 Main Street, Suite 911*
*Chester, PA 19015*
*(610) 872-7447*

# ACKNOWLEDGMENTS

Many individuals have played an important role in the development of *Emergency First Care*. Among those who have participated in, contributed to, and helped to field test it are the health professionals who have served as faculty for Emergency and Safety Programs, Inc. since 1979: Christopher Brigham, M.D., Kathleen Burke, EMT, Janice Campbell, R.N., CDR. Ken Coffland, EMT, USCG (Ret.), John Cornele, R.N., Sarah Fisher, M.D., Jim Healy, R.N.[*], Patricia Kelly-Holmes, M.D., Edward Horton, R.N., Janice Jacovini, R.N., Sal Lombardo, EMT-P, Karen March, R.N., Chip Miller, EMT-P, Doyle Moore, R.N., Shauna L. Poach, R.N., Chief Joseph Poliafico, Karen Ranieri, EMT, Bill Richard, EMT-P, Bruce Rubel, R.N., Sandra Russell, L.V.N., and Cary Wiener, Esq., R-EMT. Special contributors include: Patty Pruitt, for manuscript and layout preparation; Rosalie Morrall, for original artwork and graphics; and Bonnie McNamara, for manuscript preparation.

A special word of thanks must also go to Dr. Allen Braslow. His scholarly yet pragmatic work in the area of emergency medical educational methodology has been a guiding force in the development of *Emergency First Care*.

Particular recognition and gratitude must also go to numerous organizations for their encouragement and support and for their confidence in *Emergency First Care* over the years: Sun Transport, Inc. (Charles Ryan, M.D., Mary Swartz, Kathy Metcalf, Esq., and Dennis Kelly); Maritrans, Inc. (Dave Buchanan and

John Hihn[*]); ARCO (Judy Kambestad, Alicia Horst-Cook, Mike Delitta, Ph.D., Frank Lee, and E. H. Givens, M.D.); DuPont (Peter Walker); Eastern Airlines (Denise Noe and Joyce Montgomery); Gulf Coast Transit (Sal Litrico and Bill Fassler); Hollywood Marine, Inc. (Jim Tighe and Marsha McNorton); Marine Transport Lines (David Wood and Nick Orfanidis); Northwest Airlines (Karen Hanlon, Peter Wilander, and Katheryn Ray); Spenton Bush/Red Star Companies (Stan Chelluck and Bill Serba); Sea River Maritime, Inc. (John Gelland); Scott Paper Company (L. Luke Cellini, M.D. and Rose Morris, R.N.); Samedan Oil Corporation (Don Bullard[*], Steve Taylor, Steve Molbert, and Steve Shuman); and United Airlines (Frank Connell, Janice Northcott, Tim Cameron, and Helen Zienkievicz, R.N.).

Thanks also go to those who reviewed the manuscript: Allan Silvester, EMT-P, Mobile, AL; Dana B. Hinkley, Berlin, NH Fire Department; Captain David L. Wood, Marine Transport Lines, Inc., Weehawken, NJ; Shawn Fix, RPM, NREMT-P, Emergency Medical Consultant, Inc., Port St. Lucie, FL; Helen Zienkievicz, R.N., ANP, United Airlines, Inflight Safety, Chicago, IL; Ham Robbins, R.N. Paramedic, RENT-A-MEDIC, Readfield, ME; Gary Waites, Administrative and Emergency Training, Sante Fe, TX; and Joe Grafft, MS, EMS Specialist, State Board of Technical Colleges, St. Paul, MN.

To a number of publishing professionals at Brady/Prentice Hall whose creative talent and genius helped in bringing this book to completion, I am most grateful: Susan Katz, V.P./Publisher; Judy Streger, Marketing Manager; Julie Boddorf, Production Editor; Patrick Walsh, Managing Production Editor; Michal Heron, Managing Photography Editor; and Michael O'Neill, Photographer.

A note of thanks also goes to the principal developers and promoters of the "Make the Right Call" program: United States Fire Association, National Highway Traffic Safety Administration, and Ogilvy, Adams & Rinehart.

My heartfelt gratitude goes to my wife Margie, our daughters Julie and Kate, and my mother Vi for their endless love, support, and patience.

. . . and finally, my appreciation goes to the hundreds of men and women working on land, at sea, and in the sky who have participated in this program since 1979, and for whom *Emergency First Care* was developed.

---

[*]May they rest in peace.

# ABOUT THE AUTHOR

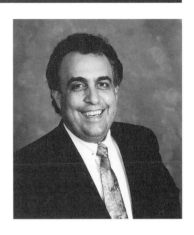

Frank J. Poliafico is founder and President of Emergency and Safety Programs, Inc., of Chester, Pennsylvania. A recognized leader in emergency medical services development, he is a graduate of the Nursing Program of Widener University (1971). Frank began his career as an emergency department nurse and was a pioneer in the development of educational programs for Emergency Medical Technicians, Paramedics, and Emergency Department Nurses, as well as non-medical personnel in a variety of work settings. From 1977–1980, he served as Director of Emergency Medical Services (EMS) for New York City; he also directed the development of emergency medical service systems in the Delaware County (Pennsylvania) and Miami areas.

Mr. Poliafico has served on numerous local, state, and national medical and health advisory committees and professional associations. He is a member of the National Nurses in Business Association, was a board member of the National Emergency Nurses Association, served on the American Medical Association Task Force on Paramedic Training Standards, and was a consultant and grant reviewer for the United States Department of Health and Education for emergency medical services funding.

In the 1970s he helped to form the Pennsylvania Emergency Health Services Council and Mid-Atlantic EMS Council and served on the executive committee of both. He has served as a consultant to the United State Surgeon General for the government publication, *The Ship's Medicine Chest and Medical Aid at Sea*, is a member of the Marine Section of the National Safety Council, and is on the planning committee of the annual Aircraft Cabin Safety Symposium presented by the Southern California Safety Institute.

Since 1980, he has been applying the advances of EMS programs to the needs of industry and government agencies on land, at sea, and in the sky. He has developed and conducted unique and creative illness and injury prevention and control training programs, nationally and internationally, for such companies and agencies as ARCO, DuPont, Singapore Airlines, EXXON, United Airlines, the F.B.I., the Massachusetts Department of Corrections, and many others.

# PART 1

## GETTING STARTED: RATIONALE, READINESS, AND RECOGNITION

Properly trained emergency medical professionals are rarely the ones who first encounter and attend to a sick or injured person's medical needs. Despite numerous improvements in the field of EMS, the outcome of medical emergencies is often determined not only by EMTs, paramedics, emergency nurses, and trauma surgeons, but also by family members, co-workers, and other individuals who usually are the first people to detect and respond to a medical emergency.

When a sudden illness or injury occurs, modern paramedic ambulances and medical centers can be 10 to 30 minutes away, if not more. Whether or not sophisticated medical services are available on-site when a medical emergency occurs, the application of simple life support procedures by properly trained and motivated non-medical personnel until professional medical help is available has proved effective in controlling the physical and fiscal complications of a serious illness or injury. Such actions, until professional help is available, will help assure the likelihood of the victim's survival.

Before you are confronted with someone who may be having a serious medical emergency and prior to providing needed life support actions:

1. Understand why your actions are so important.

2. Have a simple and effective plan to follow.

3. Believe that you can make a difference.

4. Know the indications for when to initiate your plan.

5. Determine which potentially life-threatening problems can be controlled and the status of essential body systems.

# CHAPTER 1

## INTRODUCTION TO EMERGENCY FIRST CARE

Throughout the country and the world, serious illness and injury exact a significant toll in terms of suffering, loss of life and staggering economic impact. Each day there are hundreds of people sustaining serious events:

HEART ATTACKS
INDUSTRIAL INJURIES
SUDDEN DEATHS
AUTOMOBILE FATALITIES
SLIPS AND FALLS
DIABETIC EMERGENCIES
STROKES
SEIZURES
KNIFE AND GUNSHOT WOUNDS
DROWNINGS
ETC., ETC., ETC. . . .

These calamities are not limited to any particular age, sex, race, ethnic group, socioeconomic class, or specific workplace.

## MYTHS AND MISCONCEPTIONS

"It only happens to the other guy."

**JUST THE FACTS:**
If this were true, statistically you would be at great risk because to everyone else, *you* are the other guy! Sudden injury and illness can and do happen to anyone, and you may well be the one who detects and must respond to a potentially life-threatening event.

Medical emergencies can happen at home, at work, or at play. It is therefore important that you have the confidence and ability needed to:

1. Recognize a possible medical emergency.

2. Decide to help.

3. Contact medical help.

4. Take the appropriate First Care actions.

Emergency First Care was created to help you develop the skills and confidence necessary to assist the victim of a sudden illness or accident in a reasonable and appropriate manner, until the afflicted person is in the care of medical professionals.

## SAFETY AND HEALTH FIRST

The best way to deal with a medical emergency is to PREVENT IT! Many people pride themselves on their farsightedness in having established creative retirement plans, yet they fail to remember that saving for retirement must be physical as well as fiscal. Careful attention to prudent, healthful, and safe living habits and behavior is everyone's primary responsibility.

You must take care of yourself now, not just when you are older. The fact is that due to modern medical technology and governmental safety initiatives, people are living longer than ever before. Your quality of life, i.e., how well you will live in your "golden years" is most often determined by your lifestyle and work habits today.

The message of this book is therefore very simple: **Be Healthy! Be Safe!** But just in case someone else isn't, **Be Ready!**

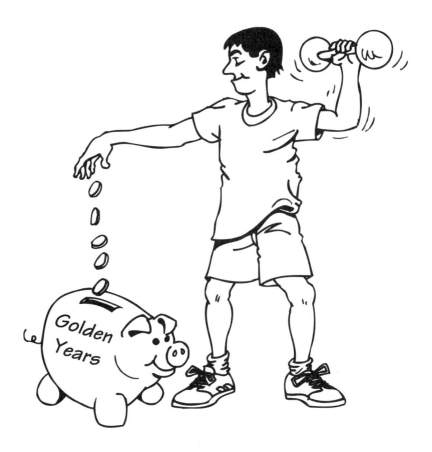

## ILLNESS AND INJURY CONTROL

Be ready to control the physical and fiscal consequences of someone's accident or illness. Medical-care costs continue to rise at an alarming rate. Hospital, legal, insurance, and doctor's fees have reached an all-time high.

A proven way to limit the economic burden of a medical crisis is to deal with the problem as early in the event as possible. If you are ready to respond immediately to someone's serious medical situation, you can often significantly reduce the overall expense of care for that person and/or the high price of litigation that frequently follows accidents, especially at work.

Reducing the fiscal risks is a benefit of Emergency First Care actions but the primary goal of this program is to minimize the *physical risks* to the victims of sudden illness and injury.

## CONTROL, NOT RESOLVE

It is not the responsibility of the First Care Giver to cure, heal, or otherwise resolve someone's medical problem. Rather, as a First Care Giver it's your role to control the emergency patient's condition as best you can. If at all possible, DON'T LET IT GET WORSE.

Because only certain physical problems can possibly be controlled outside of a sophisticated medical center, there are limits to what you can do to help an ill or injured person. Nevertheless, your actions can make a significant difference by slowing down the negative chain of events in the body of the patient.

## THE WORST THAT CAN HAPPEN: DEATH

The worst consequence of a medical emergency is for the patient to die. However, it's important to note that patients who die rarely die from the initial problem or event they sustain. Regardless of the initial diagnosis, the leading cause of death and most common factor in all deaths is usually COMPLICATIONS.

Cardiac patients usually don't die from heart attacks, they die from the physical, chemical, and electrical complications that follow damage to the heart muscle. Burn victims rarely, if ever, die from their burns. They die from complications of breathing, fluid imbalance, and infection occurring in the minutes to months following their burns.

### The Number One Complication

The most common controllable complication is a condition known as *shock*. The highly technical definition of shock is "the condition in which the cardiovascular system fails to provide sufficient oxygenated blood to all the tissues of the body." But our definition is much simpler and to the point: *SHOCK = SHUTDOWN!*

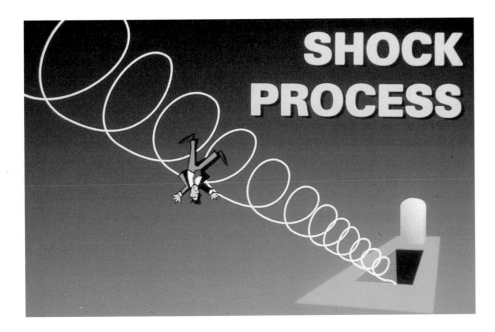

Shock is a bodily defense system. It's the body's response to the brain's recognition of a serious (or potentially serious) problem in or insult to the body. During shock the brain sends messages that systematically begin to shut down or significantly limit the function of all body systems not immediately essential to life. But shock can quickly become out of control and begin to also shut down some of the body's systems that are essential to life.

In essence, shock puts the body in a downward spiral as the brain tries to conserve its most vital resource, oxygen. There's not much a First Care Giver can or should do to control the shutdown and loss of function of the digestive system, musculoskeletal system, or circulation to the skin—all important functions within the human body.

## WHAT CAN BE DONE

The First Care Giver can, however, assist the most essential body systems in doing their job. The part of the body most responsible for life is the brain. The organ systems and structures most essential to the function of the brain are:

> BREATHING SYSTEM—LUNGS AND RELATED TUBES
> CIRCULATORY SYSTEM—HEART, VESSELS, AND BLOOD
> CERVICAL SPINE—SPINAL COLUMN AND CORD

By helping airway, breathing, circulation, and the spine, you can enhance the flow of oxygen to the brain. You can help control the shock process which, if left unchecked, will usually result in the end of life.

## SUPPORT LIFE

It is therefore your role as a First Care Giver to support life. By helping the body's most essential functions, i.e., AIRWAY, BREATHING, CIRCULATION, and SPINE, do their jobs, you can help to control the leading cause of death, complications.

## WHAT'S YOUR TITLE NOW?

First Care Giver is your description, not your title, at the time of a medical emergency. Actually, unless you're an emergency medical professional, your title in society has little to do with expectations or actions at the time of a medical emergency.

We all have many titles in life: Mom, Dad, Seafarer, Flight Attendant, Officer, Electrician, Secretary, etc. These titles indicate our roles and important functions in our families, communities, or workplaces.

No title is necessary to help someone who is having a medical emergency, no matter where you are or what your vocation. Your responsibility is to support life by giving Emergency First Care. It is the purpose of this book to help you do it!

## CERTIFICATION VS. CAPABILITIES

There are numerous regulatory agencies and professional associations requiring that certain individuals receive training in immediate emergency care actions (first aid) and/or cardiopulmonary resuscitation (CPR). If you are in a profession or occupation that requires such training you will have to complete a course or program approved by the appropriate regulatory body. You will then be "certified" that you completed the required training.

To give someone Emergency First Care you need only knowledge and skills, not a current card or certificate. The only degree needed to give immediate life support is a "High Degree of Self-Confidence."

# CHAPTER 2

## THE EMERGENCY MEDICAL SITUATION: FOUR GOLDEN RULES

What if . . . ?

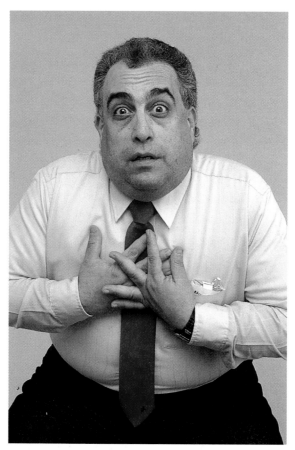

Somebody suddenly grabs his chest . . .

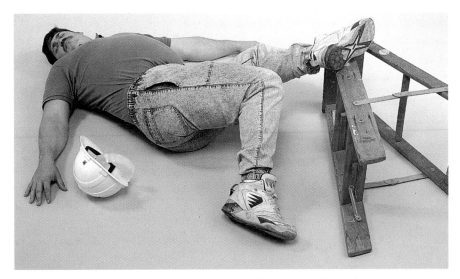

You find someone lying at the bottom of a ladder bleeding from his head . . .

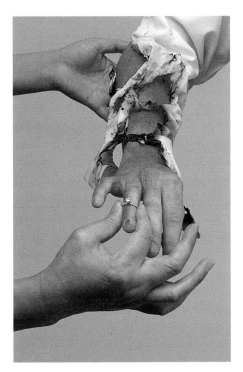

Someone burns her arm . . .

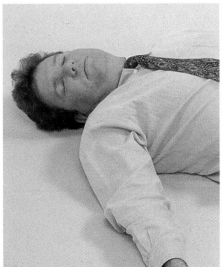

Somebody is unconscious . . .

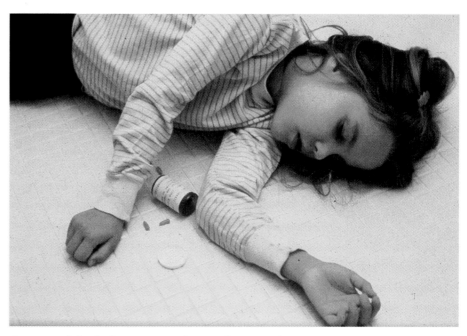

Or one of the kids gets into the medicine cabinet. . . .

These are all situations where you will probably hear yourself say, "Uh-oh!" That's your emotions motivating you to take action. To do the right things you need a plan to follow.

The Emergency First Care Golden Rules provide a well defined plan and rationale for dealing with medical emergencies in a controlled and organized way.

RULE #1:   SURVIVE
RULE #2:   DO NO HARM
RULE #3:   GET HELP
RULE #4:   SUPPORT LIFE

## THE FIRST GOLDEN RULE: SURVIVE

## PROTECT YOURSELF

Emergencies often produce physical hazards. Your first and number one concern must be for yourself. When you sense that someone has sustained a medical emergency, your first action must be to insure your own safety.

CTA = CHECK THE AREA

Take a look around. Don't let whatever happened to the victim happen to you. You must protect yourself. The first priority for all emergency responders is self-survival!

Is there a fire? Can it easily be controlled by a fire extinguisher? If not, get out and call the fire department!

Is there an exposed live electrical wire? Stay out of the area. If you can, find the right circuit breaker and turn the power off. Or find some nonconductive item like a dry wooden stick to disengage the wire from the victim. If you can't, find an electrician, maintenance person, or rescue worker.

Was the injury caused by another person? Is that person still there, still dangerous? Call the police.

Is there an accident in the middle of the highway? *Before* you get near the car, stop the flow of traffic. Don't let yourself become injured. **YOU CAN'T BE OF ANY HELP TO ANYONE IF YOU BECOME A VICTIM.**

## KNOW YOURSELF

Know what you can do and what you can't do. If you can't swim, don't jump into the water to save someone. Is there smoke or fumes? You can't breathe in smoke, fumes, and super-heated air, so don't run into a burning building. If it is available and you are trained to do so, find and don a breathing apparatus or—STAY AWAY!

*Walk, don't run!* Running is a frequent mistake that many people make at the time of a medical emergency. Don't run. You can fall. You can get hurt. Walk briskly, but don't use up your energy or your breath by running. You might need to share your breath with the victim.

### Protect Against Catching Things

The risk of getting AIDS, hepatitis, or any other disease by touching another person is very slim. Nevertheless, you should be careful. If you can, put on latex gloves or create a barrier of some sort between the patient's body fluids and your skin.

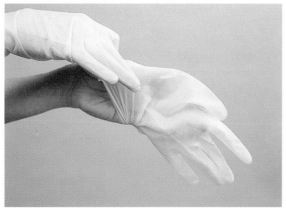

Gently pull latex gloves over each hand. Be careful not to touch your face, mouth, or eyes once bodily fluids are on your gloves.

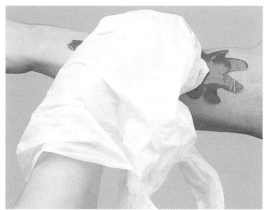

If gloves are not available, use trash bag or shirt as a barrier between your hands and the patient's body fluids.

There is a proper and safe way to remove contaminated gloves.

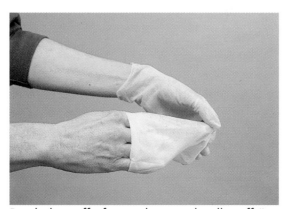

Pinch the cuff of one glove and pull it off "inside out." (Hold it in gloved hand.)

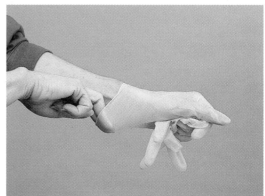

Slide your bare fingers under the cuff of the second glove and pull it off "inside out" over the first glove.

When the emergency is over, wash your hands. Public health officials are generally unanimous in their position that frequent and proper hand washing is one of the best ways to reduce your risk of contracting most infectious diseases. Catching things (viral or bacterial) is often a hand-to-mouth event. Effective hand washing cannot be accomplished in a ceremonial or ritualistic "anointing" of the fingers with water.

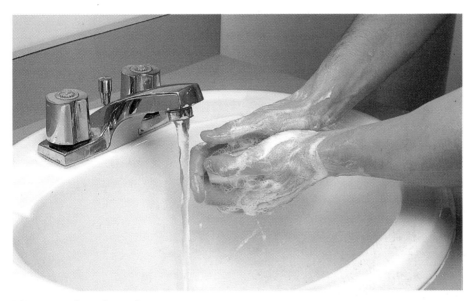

Wet your hands under warm running water.

Lather up with soap.

Briskly rub hands and fingers together for at least 15–30 seconds.

Rinse under warm running water.

Dry thoroughly.

Use antiseptic towelettes if soap and water are not available.

## EMOTIONAL SURVIVAL

### You will have emotions.

Medical emergencies produce *emotions*. You're human; you're going to feel a lot of emotions when you are suddenly faced with a medical emergency. Fear, anger, embarrassment, and sadness are all normal. Emotions are neither right nor wrong. They are a part of life. They actually serve a very valuable function in an emergency: They are energies in the mind that motivate you to take action.

### Control showing your emotional responses.

Crying, yelling, frantic behavior or staring off into space are all responses that emotions can generate. Your emotions and emotional responses can keep you from thinking clearly. The more intense your emotions, the less logical you are.

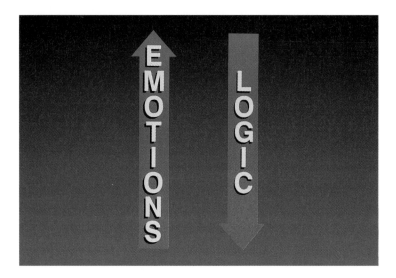

Also, emotions are contagious. The patient and any bystanders will have enough problems dealing with their own emotions; they don't need to see yours.

### Panic is loss of control.

Perhaps the most common emotional response produced by a medical emergency is panic. Panic is not an emotion, it is a mental response. Panic is fear with nothing to do! Fear is OK; it drives you into action. Panic is not OK; it paralyzes you.
YOU CAN'T CONTROL HAVING EMOTIONS. BUT YOU CAN CONTROL SHOWING THEM!

## Channel emotional energy.

To control showing your emotions, start by taking a deep breath. Then channel those emotions into doing something. The best way to control showing your emotions is to GIVE YOURSELF SOMETHING TO DO. The best thing to do is focus on your PLAN: ABCS CARE.

You must help **A**irway, **B**reathing, **C**irculation, and **S**pine to function as best they can under the circumstances and until medical help arrives, as you **C**ommunicate, **A**void harm, **R**e-examine, and **E**ncourage.

## After the emergency: Ventilate.

An important part of your personal survival will be to express your suppressed emotions after the emergency is over. The professionals call it "post traumatic stress syndrome." You've been through something that doesn't happen every day, and to handle that situation you had to keep a lid on your emotions. Suppressed emotions can eventually surface weeks, months, or even years later as a host of mental and physical ailments and symptoms.

As soon as feasible after the emergency situation has ended, "ventilate" your feelings. After your response to a crisis, it's OK and normal to have feelings of guilt, fear, or sadness, but it's not OK to "keep 'em in." Get them out of your system. Talk about it, write about it, have a "debriefing session" with friends or co-workers.

Be careful, however: Do not use alcohol or drugs to "control" these feelings. Chemical substances will only help you further suppress your emotions, very likely intensifying and prolonging any unpleasant feelings and causing more serious physical and mental consequences.

## THE SECOND GOLDEN RULE: DO NO HARM

## DON'T MOVE THE BODY OR ITS PARTS

Don't do any more damage than the accident or illness has already caused.

Don't move the person or her body parts unless you have a very good reason. Before you move anyone, ask yourself,

"WHY?" Then ask yourself, "WHY?" Then, once more, ask yourself, **"WHY?"**

If there is a good reason, you may have to move the patient. Someone lying face down in his own vomit can't breathe. Turn him over. If a building is on fire, pull the victim out. But unless you have a very good reason, leave the victim in the position you find her until help is available.

## DON'T PRACTICE "CREATIVE MEDICINE"

No one expects you to be a miracle worker . . . to do a tracheotomy with your ballpoint pen, to start someone's heart with your car battery, or to do open heart surgery with your pocket knife.

## APPEARANCE IS IMPORTANT

No one expects you to dress or look like a doctor, nurse, or medical professional. However, your appearance is extremely important to the patient. You must appear COMPETENT and CONFIDENT. You must give the appearance that YOU CAN DO IT. Your concern and appropriate actions will communicate a sense of confidence and competence to the victim.

## AVOID THE TRAP—DON'T MAKE A DIAGNOSIS

It's OK not to know.

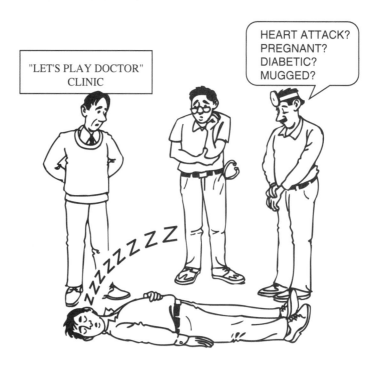

Suppose the patient is clutching his chest. Is it a heart attack? Is it indigestion? Or did the person just receive a tax bill? You don't really know. And it's OK not to know.

It's NOT your job to find out "what's wrong and why." It's NOT your role to "remedy the situation." It's NOT your place to "cure" the patient. It's NOT your job to make a "diagnosis."

It IS your role as an Emergency First Care Giver to check the ABCS and make 'em the best they can be—that is, to **SUPPORT LIFE**! Does the victim have an airway? Is the victim breathing? Is the victim bleeding? Don't waste time worrying about why. What is important is that you summon help and safely **SUPPORT LIFE** until help arrives.

## THE THIRD GOLDEN RULE: GET HELP

## YOU ARE NOT ALONE

You may be the first person to detect and respond to a medical emergency, but you are not the only one who will have an impact on the outcome. You are not expected to cure the ill person nor heal her ills. It is quite simply your responsibility to control and minimize complications until professional medical care is available.

### Know Your Resources

At your work location there may be an organized Emergency Response Team—alert them. At home, solicit and direct the help of family or neighbors.

Ask other bystanders who may be present for help and assistance. Above all, know how to activate your community's EMS system and MAKE THE RIGHT CALL.

### The Golden Hour

Comprehensive Emergency Medical Systems, referred to as EMS or 911 services, have been established in nearly every city and town. EMS is a team of highly trained, very dedicated and well-equipped dispatchers, emergency medical technicians (EMTs), paramedics, nurses, and physicians. These medical professionals can often work modern-day miracles, especially if they can provide care to a victim during the first "Golden Hour" following an illness or accident.

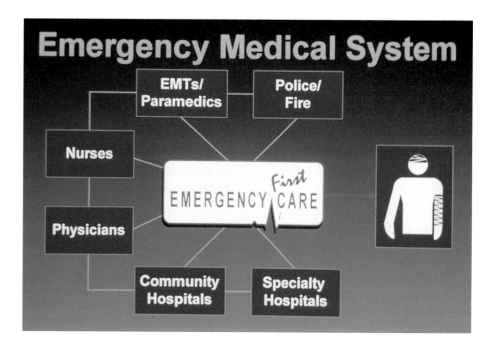

## The Silver Minutes

Sadly, however, these marvelous community EMS services are frequently useless to a suddenly ill or seriously injured person. For highly sophisticated ambulances, emergency departments, and trauma, burn care, and cardiac care centers to be of any value at all, the patient must arrive alive! For a "Golden Hour" opportunity to occur, the first person to detect a potentially life-threatening problem must do something in the precious first "Silver Minutes" to help keep life present. That something is:

1. Recognize that there may be a problem.

2. Protect yourself.

3. MAKE THE RIGHT CALL.

4. Until help arrives . . . follow the ABCS CARE plan of LIFE SUPPORT!

| A | B | C | S | | C | A | R | E |
|---|---|---|---|---|---|---|---|---|
| i | r | i | p | | o | v | e | n |
| r | e | r | i | | m | o | e | c |
| w | a | c | n | | m | i | x | o |
| a | t | u | e | | u | d | a | u |
| y | h | l | | | n | | m | r |
| | i | a | | | i | H | i | a |
| | n | t | | | c | a | n | g |
| | g | i | | | a | r | e | e |
| | | o | | | t | m | | |
| | | n | | | e | | | |

## THE ESSENCE OF LIFE

Philosophers and poets have for centuries explored and expounded on the meaning of life. Biologically, however, the continuation of a human life can be simply defined. As long as the brain receives and utilizes oxygen, human life is sustained. The essence of life is, therefore, "Oxygen to the brain" or, to quote Miami Beach EMS pioneer J. P. Healy, "Juice to the squash."

Despite its many marvels, complex biochemical processes, and creative talents, the functions of the human body most essential to maintaining life are the workings and interactions of the BRAIN, HEART, and LUNGS. By helping these organs and their respective parts do their job in an ill or injured person, a First Care Provider can truly help keep life present until professional medical care is available.

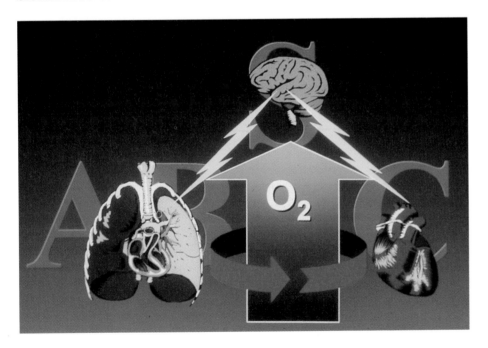

## THE PROCESS OF DEATH

To better appreciate LIFE SUPPORT it is necessary to understand DEATH.

The end of each human life is inevitable. However, death is seldom if ever instantaneous; it is instead a well-defined process that can be slowed down and often averted for many years.

"He dropped dead."
"Her time was up."
"They were killed instantly."

**JUST THE FACTS:**

Many myths and misconceptions like these have existed for years. People don't just drop dead; rarely if ever are they killed instantly. Despite statements to the contrary, most people actually believe that their "time is up" only after they have exhausted all technological and/or spiritual tools at their disposal.

## Defining Death

The usual progression of death is:

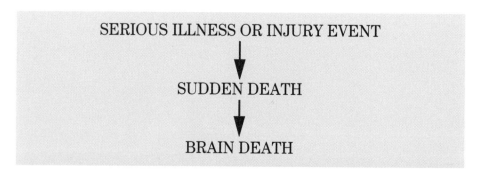

SERIOUS ILLNESS OR INJURY EVENT

↓

SUDDEN DEATH

↓

BRAIN DEATH

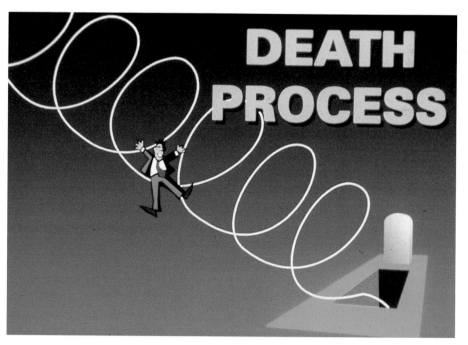

A serious illness or injury event is one where, without outside intervention, damaged body organs and systems will interfere with and/or not be able to help provide oxygen to the brain.

"Sudden death" means that heart action and breathing have stopped. However, "brain death" (or biological death) does not occur until the brain itself is no longer able to function. If nothing is done to slow down the process, brain death will usually occur within 8–10 minutes after "sudden death."

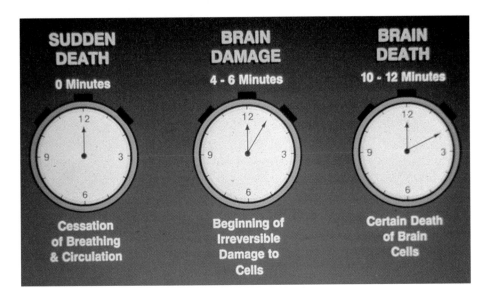

| SUDDEN DEATH | BRAIN DAMAGE | BRAIN DEATH |
| --- | --- | --- |
| 0 Minutes | 4 - 6 Minutes | 10 - 12 Minutes |
| Cessation of Breathing & Circulation | Beginning of Irreversible Damage to Cells | Certain Death of Brain Cells |

## SUPPORTING LIFE

Life support actions can affect the progression of serious illness or injury to "sudden death." Even once "sudden death" occurs, life support action can still temporarily retard "brain death." You can, therefore, significantly slow down the process of death.

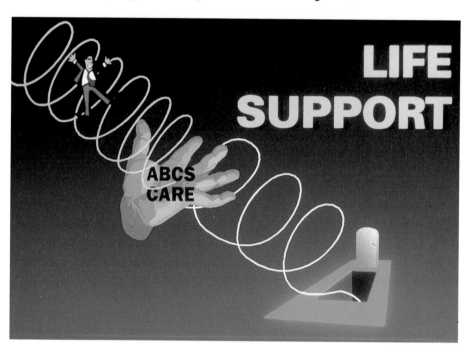

By helping the Airway, Breathing, Circulation, and Spine function the best they can under the circumstances of a serious illness or injury, you can make a dramatic difference in whether someone survives an emergency event and its complications.

# CHAPTER 3

## PATIENT EXAMINATION

## WHEN IS EMERGENCY FIRST CARE NEEDED?

How do you know when you are facing an emergency medical situation? The answer will usually come to you directly from your KSO: Keen Sense of the Obvious. It is virtually impossible for someone to be critically ill or injured and look fine. Several key indicators will trigger your KSO and alert you that a medical emergency may be present.

### Mechanism of Injury

When someone experiences a rapid deceleration event (that is, a body is in motion and abruptly stops against some fixed object, or an object is in motion and abruptly stops against—or in—a body) he may well have sustained a serious injury.

Perhaps the most classic deceleration event is someone's unbelted body striking the windshield and dashboard when a car going 40 miles per hour stops abruptly. Other examples of deceleration are a fall from a ladder or down the stairs. However, even collapsing to the floor from a standing position can potentially cause serious harm. Auto, sledding, and driving accidents, as well as slips and falls, are the most common Mechanisms of Injury (MOI).

### Significant Complaint

Someone describing an unusual pain or sensation that suddenly occurs in his body may be experiencing a medical emergency. Chest pain or discomfort, numbness in an arm, or a pounding headache, if untypical for that person, may well be an indication of a serious problem.

## Change in Appearance, Speech, or Color

Other indicators of an emergency medical problem are: When someone's speech suddenly becomes slurred or confused. When her skin color changes dramatically, becoming pale or blue. When her mental status is altered, becoming confused, unharacteristically irritable, or unresponsive.

When your KSO is alerted, you have to do something. But before you do something inappropriate or ineffective, take a closer look to determine what problems are possibly controllable.

## WHEN KSO SAYS "UH-OH"

When your KSO recognizes:

- A mechanism of injury
- Someone's significant complaint
- A dramatic change in someone's physical appearance

your decision to act will need to be followed by your Emergency First Care plan.

### RULE #1: SURVIVE

Check the area (CTA) for potential hazards to yourself. Eliminate or neutralize these hazards, if possible. If body fluids are present, put on latex gloves, if available (or use a barrier of some sort).

### RULE # 2: DO NO HARM

Don't move an ill or injured person's body or parts unless absolutely necessary. Don't "play doctor" by attempting to determine a diagnosis, but do look for life-threatening problems about which you can do something.

## RULE # 3: GET HELP

Call out to nearby family or coworkers. Notify the Emergency Response Team (if at work). As soon as possible, MAKE THE RIGHT CALL (EMS).

## RULE # 4: SUPPORT LIFE

Help maintain life by assisting Airway, Breathing, Circulation, and Spine to be as efficient as possible.

Before you can support life, however, you need to determine specific ABCS needs. This is done with a simple but rapid examination known as the Quik Chek.

## LOOKING FOR CONTROLLABLE PROBLEMS

Sometimes your eyes and your mind play tricks on you; what you see really isn't what it may at first appear to be. For example, the lines in the figure appear to be different lengths, but further examination—generally with a ruler of some sort—reveals that they are the same size.

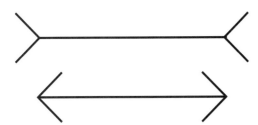

In what appears to be a possible medical emergency, the sights, sounds, and emotions of the moment can also be misleading. If you rely on your first impressions, you can miss significant problems that you may be well able to control and prevent from becoming more serious complications. You therefore need a "ruler," a way to accurately measure the presence of life and to establish priorities to support life.

# THE QUIK CHEK

Once your safety and the patient's are assured, begin looking for life-threatening problems and complications for which you can provide assistance. In Emergency First Care the measuring tool or "ruler" to determine a person's emergency care needs is called a Quik Chek.

Doing a Quik Chek is as simple as ABCS. You will use these steps to examine the body's structures and functions most essential to life:

> **A**IRWAY
> **B**REATHING
> **C**IRCULATION
> **S**PINE

## Position the Patient

The patient will need to be in a proper position for you to examine him. If someone is face down and unresponsive, it will be difficult (if not impossible) to do a Quik Chek.

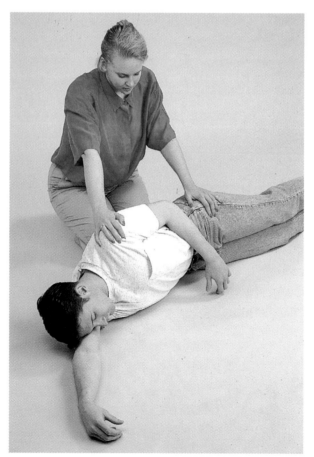

One person doing log roll.

Because of the possibility of spine injury you are going to have to reposition him very carefully. The preferred method for repositioning an unresponsive face-down person is called the *log roll*. By moving the body as a unit and keeping the head, neck, and back in a straight line there is less risk of doing additional damage to the spinal column or spinal cord.

You can accomplish a log roll by yourself; however, the more people you have to help you accomplish this maneuver, the safer it will be for the patient.

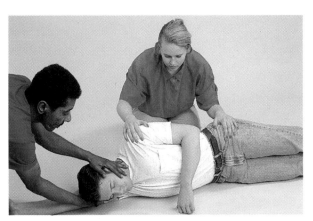

Two-person log roll.

## QUIK CHEK AIRWAY

### Helpful Background Information

The airway is one of the simplest yet most important structures in the human body. Through this passage, the chemical most essential to life, oxygen, flows into the lungs. From the lungs it is absorbed into the blood and then circulated to the brain and other parts of the body by the pumping of the heart.

Also known as the trachea or windpipe, the airway is nearly an inch in diameter and four to five inches long in adults (proportionally smaller in children). It is made up of semicircular cartilage rings; thin, smooth muscles; and a delicate mucus membrane lining. Located at its upper end are the vocal cords and a protective "trap door"-like flap of tissue known as the epiglottis.

At the lower end the airway branches into two tubes (the bronchi) which lead to the left and right lungs. Airway blockage is a major threat to life. The most common cause of obstruction of the airway is the tongue "falling back" against the opening to the windpipe. The tongue is attached to the lower jaw. When someone is unconscious the jaw relaxes, which can result in the tongue going backwards.

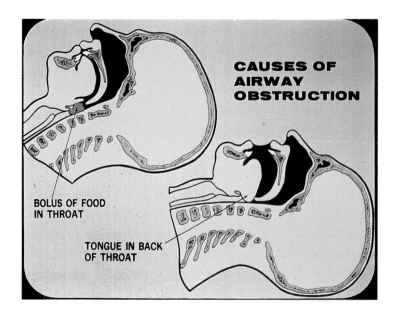

CAUSES OF AIRWAY OBSTRUCTION

BOLUS OF FOOD IN THROAT

TONGUE IN BACK OF THROAT

Another controllable airway problem is choking. Choking occurs when food or some other object wedges on top of or underneath the protective flap of tissue at the entrance to the windpipe. When someone is choking, she will not be able to talk or make any verbal sounds. If someone doesn't respond verbally, his airway is potentially blocked by something.

## Determine Airway Problems

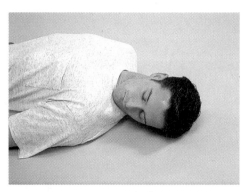

Unconsciousness and chin position are the major indications of a possible airway threat.

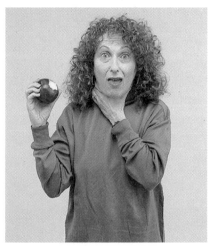

The tongue is the most common cause of airway obstruction.

Signs of choking can include:
- Hands at throat
- Food being consumed
- Change in color
- Look of terror
- Inability to speak

# Airway Quik Chek Summary

❏ UNCONSCIOUS
❏ CHIN POSITION
❏ SIGNS OF CHOKING

## QUIK CHEK BREATHING

### Helpful Background Information

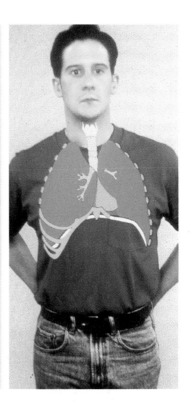

Breathing brings air (containing oxygen) into the body and expels unused air and waste byproducts (largely carbon dioxide) from the body. Several body structures and organs are responsible for the breathing process. Most notable are two soft, spongy, elastic tissue organs, the lungs.

Each lung is enclosed in an airtight sac. When fully expanded, the lungs can hold nearly five quarts of air. Generally only a half quart is exchanged in each normal breath.

Most important to the actual process of breathing are the diaphragm, a muscle across the bottom of the chest cavity, and the smaller muscles between the ribs. When the diaphragm relaxes it moves down, lowering pressure in the lungs and allowing them to take in air. As it contracts the diaphragm moves up, raising pressure and expelling air from the lungs. During breathing the muscles in the area of the ribs also play a part in the process by enlarging the chest cavity upward and outward.

### Determine Breathing Problems

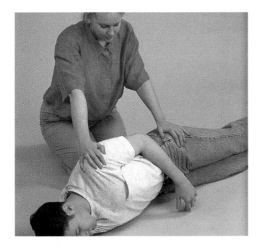

As chin lift is maintained, look and feel for chest and/or belly movement. Listen for breath sounds from mouth and nose as you feel for air flow against your outer ear. Look, listen, and feel for at least five seconds to be sure of your findings.

## Breathing Quik Chek Summary

- ❏ LOOK
- ❏ LISTEN
- ❏ FEEL

## Getting Help

In any medical emergency, professional medical help should be summoned as soon as possible. However, every situation is different. Here are some general guidelines you can use for calling professional medical help:

1. Whenever possible, send someone else to call for help so you can stay with and attend to the patient. Be sure to have that person come back and tell you if and when help is coming.

2. If you are alone with the patient, if emergency medical services are available in a matter of minutes, and if you believe the situation is serious (the patient is unresponsive, or not breathing), go call for help, even if it means leaving the patient. Once help is on the way, you should provide life support as best you can until medical professionals arrive.

3. If professional medical help is not readily available (aboard a ship, on a plane, in the wilderness, etc.), provide support for the ABCS. Use your judgment to decide when you will have to leave the patient to go for help.

4. If the patient is unresponsive and there is no obvious mechanism of injury, before you go to call for help, position the patient on his side to avoid airway problems.

## QUIK CHEK CIRCULATION

### Helpful Background Information

The circulatory system is made up of three parts: the pump, the pipes, and the fluid. Its primary purpose is to transport oxygen and other essential chemicals to the brain and other body tissues.

---

**IMPORTANT POINT**

In general, as you determine the lack of ABCS during the Quik Chek, you should deal with that problem immediately. However, if you find that someone is unresponsive and not breathing, stop and call EMS immediately (if available) before initiating life support or continuing your Quik Chek. If possible, have someone else place the call; if not, you must "MAKE THE RIGHT CALL" yourself. Then continue the Quik Chek and needed life support.

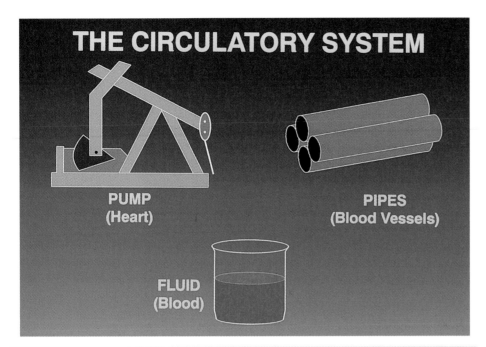

# THE CIRCULATORY SYSTEM

**PUMP**
(Heart)

**PIPES**
(Blood Vessels)

**FLUID**
(Blood)

The heart is a flexible, hollow organ not much larger than a fist, located just behind the breastbone. As the brain signals, the heart squeezes and relaxes in a steady rhythmic fashion, creating pressure that moves the blood in the arteries and veins throughout the body.

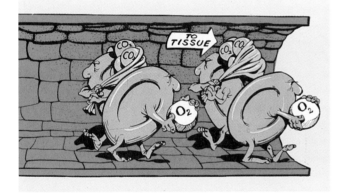

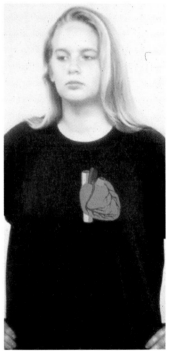

About 12 pints of blood fill literally thousands of miles of blood vessels in the adult body. Of the blood's several functions, the most significant is carrying oxygen molecules throughout the body and especially to the brain.

## IMPORTANT POINT

Don't use your thumbs. Never feel both sides of neck at once. Practice taking a neck pulse on yourself and others.

## Determine Circulation Problems

Place your middle finger on the Adam's Apple at the center of the throat. Slide these two fingers into muscle groove at side of neck and feel for rhythmic pulsations.

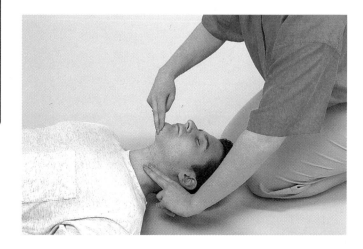

Look for obvious serious bleeding and try to determine its source.

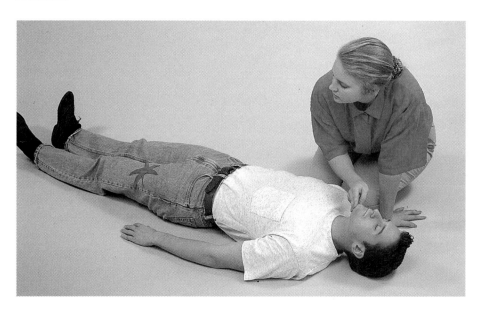

## Circulation Quik Chek Summary

❑ FEEL FOR A PULSE
❑ LOOK FOR BLEEDING

# QUIK CHEK SPINE

## Helpful Background Information

The human brain is the "boss" organ. It is the center of thought, emotion, and memory; it controls all voluntary and involuntary body functions. It is without question the most remarkable and complicated part of the body.

However, for the brain to perform its complex function of sending and receiving messages to and from other body organs and systems it needs a communication link. This link is provided by the spinal cord.

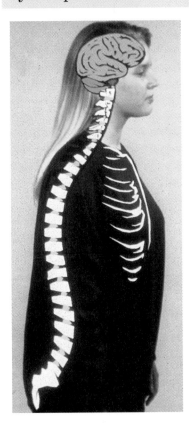

The spinal cord is literally an extension of the brain, with thousands of smaller "nerve lines" extending off it to all parts of the body. It is enclosed in the spinal column, which is made of irregularly shaped bones stacked one on top of the other.

This creates a simple but sturdy structure to protect the very delicate spinal cord (which has about the consistency of cold butter). However, if these bones are broken or shifted out of place by injury, they can severely damage the spinal cord.

The skull, which surrounds and encloses the brain, is very durable. Often a blow to the head will cause no damage to the skull or brain but may be transmitted to the very delicate bones in the neck. Generally, signs of a head injury indicate a possible spine injury.

Of all the millions of messages transmitted from the brain via the spinal cord, the two most important to sustaining life are for the heart to beat and the lungs to breathe. Damage to the neck area can interrupt or impair these vital messages. Therefore, injured persons must be carefully examined to determine the possibility of a spinal column or spinal cord injury.

## TYPES OF INJURIES TO NECK AND SPINE

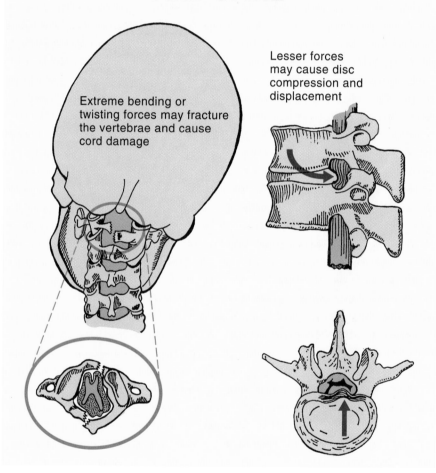

Extreme bending or twisting forces may fracture the vertebrae and cause cord damage

Lesser forces may cause disc compression and displacement

## Determine Spine Problems

Look for indications of a Mechanism of Injury (MOI). Note: Anyone found on the ground or floor and unconscious should be considered to have sustained an MOI!

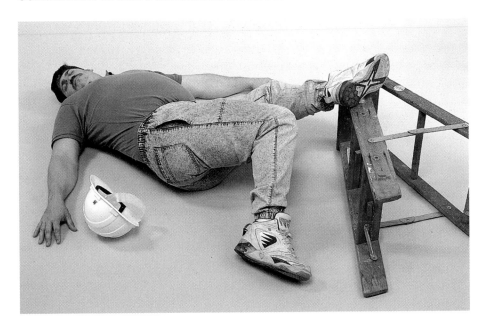

Without moving the head, gently feel the back of the neck for pain, tenderness, or obvious deformity.

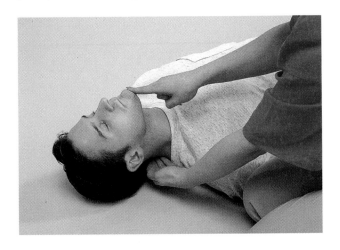

Gently drag your fingers over the head, feeling for evidence of bumps, wounds, or pain. Look for blood or clear fluid coming from ears and/or nose.

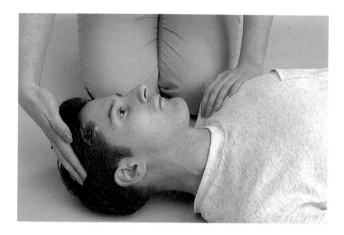

Ask a conscious victim to wiggle his fingers and ask if any unusual sensations are present (numbness, "pins and needles," or pain).

## IMPORTANT POINT

If you find any one of the above indications of spine injury, STOP! Don't bother checking for any others. Consider your victim to have a spine injury and provide appropriate support until medical help arrives.

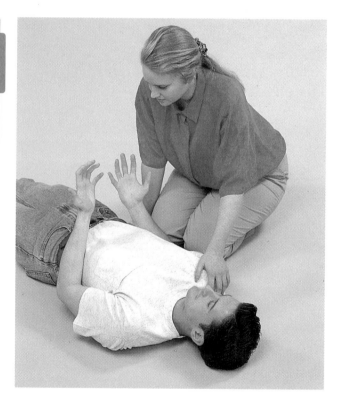

## Spine Quik Chek Summary

> ❏ MECHANISM OF INJURY
> ❏ NECK PAIN OR DEFORMITY
> ❏ HEAD INJURY
> ❏ LIMB SENSATION

## WHY DO A QUIK CHEK?

1. Gain control of yourself and the situation.

2. Gain the confidence of the sick or injured person and by-standers.

3. Discover life-threatening problems that can be controlled.

4. Set priorities for life support.

5. Be able to provide information to medical professionals.

## The Results of a Quik Chek

The performance of a Quik Chek examination at the time of a perceived medical emergency will result in one of three determinations:

1. The ill or injured person is alive, but something is wrong.

2. The person is definitely dead and beyond help.

3. The ill or injured person has suffered "sudden death."

If the ill or injured person is breathing and has a pulse, you will need to support the processes of Airway, Breathing, Circulation, and Spine until help arrives. Determining that someone is dead and beyond help is a most unpleasant consideration. In obvious situations such as decapitation, charring of entire body, or decomposition, there is nothing you or anyone can do to help.

If, however, someone has no heartbeat, is not breathing, and has none of the signs of permanent death, you should presume that it's "sudden death" and support life by providing Airway, Breathing, and Circulation with CPR (Cardiopulmonary Rescusitation) until help arrives.

# FIRST CARE CHEKSHEET™

## "QUIK CHEK"™

✓ **Check The Area**

☐ Hazards

☐ Latex Gloves

✓ **Do No Harm**

☐ Responsiveness?

✓ **Call Out for Help**

☐ Body Position

A – Airway

☐ Chin Position

☐ Signs of Obstruction

B – Breathing

☐ Look

☐ Listen

☐ Feel

✓ **Seek Medical Help??**

C – Circulation

☐ Pulse

☐ Bleeding

S – Spine

☐ Mechanism of Injury

☐ Neck

☐ Head

☐ Limb Sensation

✓ **Support Life**

✓ **Make the Right Call (EMS)???**

# *You can do it!*

# PART 2

## LIFE SUPPORT FOR THE SERIOUSLY ILL OR INJURED

When you recognize (KSO) that someone may be having a medical emergency, your plan is:

1. **Check The Area**
   - Insure your own safety
   - Put on latex gloves

2. Do No Harm
   - Don't move the body or its parts
   - Don't make a diagnosis
   - Quik Chek for controllable life-threatening problems

3. Send or Call for Help
   - Notify the Emergency Response Team (if at work)
   - Make the Right Call (EMS)

4. Support Life
   - ABCS: Presence is not productivity!
   - Help . . . Airway
           Breathing
           Circulation
           Spine . . . **Be the Best They Can Be!**

Through effective life support you can slow down and minimize the process of shock and enhance the body's efforts to survive.

# CHAPTER 4

## SUPPORT AIRWAY

Opening and maintaining a person's airway is always the first patient care action in the life support process. Without an open air passage, oxygen cannot enter the body. Several important and related actions may be necessary.

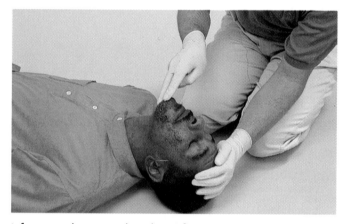

Lift up and out on the chin (if unresponsive).

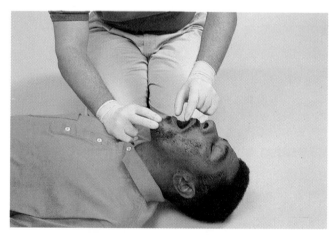

Clear the mouth of any foreign matter (food, gum, loose dentures).

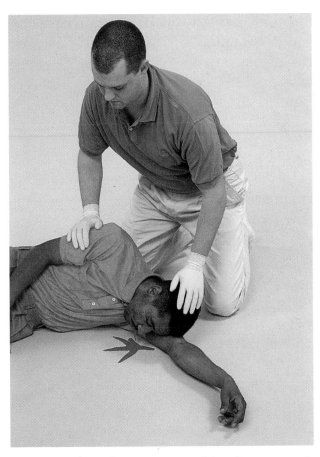

Place on side to drain secretions (blood, vomit, etc.).

## SPECIAL AIRWAY SUPPORT SITUATIONS

If you have a suspicion of head and neck injury (as in the case of someone who fell), or if an individual sustains severe facial trauma (as could result from a face striking the windshield in an auto accident), you will need to exercise special care in the support of a patient's airway.

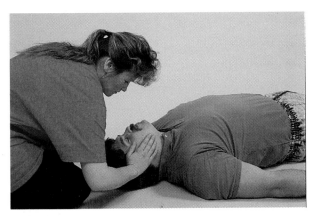

Perform a "modified jaw thrust."

This jaw thrust procedure has the added benefit of allowing the rescuer to simultaneously immobilize the cervical spine area by holding the patient's head in a fixed position. This is important because often the trauma sustained in severe facial injury can produce serious damage to the cervical spine area.

## Exception to Airway Support

An exception to the priority and procedures for airway support is for a person having a grand mal seizure. If a person's body suddenly stiffens and begins to shake dramatically, an electrical malfunction in the brain known as a seizure or convulsion is occurring.

---

### MYTHS AND MISCONCEPTIONS

"Place something—a spoon, bite stick, or some other object—in a seizuring patient's mouth so she won't swallow her tongue."

**JUST THE FACTS:**

It is impossible for someone to swallow his/her tongue. The tongue is attached to the lower jaw, which makes it impossible to be swallowed without also swallowing the jaw and lower plate! Someone having a seizure may bite his tongue, but once the jaw and face muscles stiffen (as they do during a grand mal seizure) there is nothing you can do to move or open a tightly clenched jaw without running the risk of causing serious harm.

---

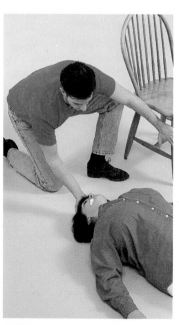

*During a seizure*

- Help patient safely to floor.
- Move furniture or objects (if possible).
- Put NOTHING IN PATIENT'S MOUTH.
- Do not restrain or hold patient down.

*After convulsion stops*

- Maintain chin lift.
- Position on side (if "frothing at mouth" or secretions occur).
- Provide ABCS CARE.
- Get medical help.

# FOOD OR FOREIGN MATTER OBSTRUCTION

## Helpful Background Information

After the tongue, the most common cause of airway obstruction is food. Because this emergency often occurs in restaurants, and because the patient's problem is often mistaken for a heart attack, this episode is commonly referred to as "Café Coronary."

Food or any other matter lodged in the back of the throat or actually in the windpipe is the one medical emergency that is completely resolvable. When someone is choking, the airway structures go into spasm (in an attempt to keep the object from going deeper), but this also prevents air from entering or leaving the lungs. However, because we never exhale completely, there is always air remaining in the body. By forcing that air out of the lungs through the airway (by pushing in and up on the diaphragm muscle), the obstruction is literally popped out like a cork from a bottle.

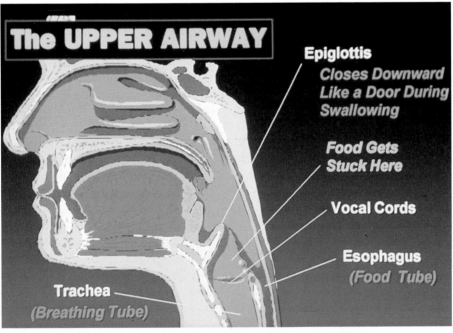

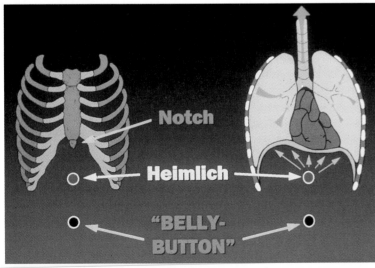

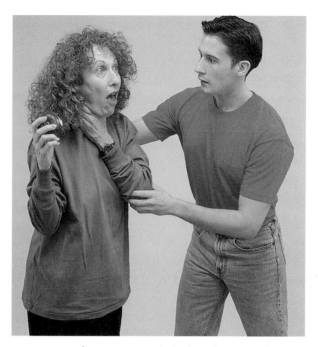

Determine if person needs help (clasping throat, looks scared, makes no sound).

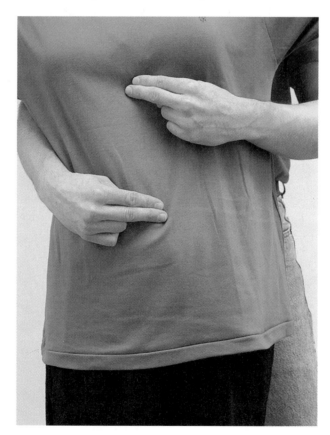

From behind standing victim, find "landmarks": notch at bottom of her breastbone and belly button.

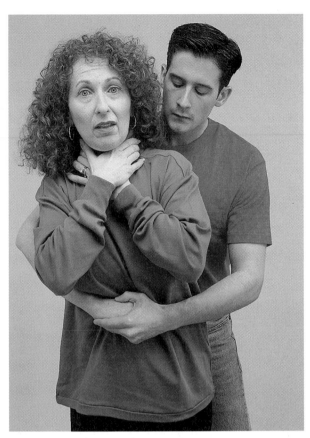

Place your fist and other hand on abdomen (half-way between these "landmarks") and thrust up and in repeatedly until obstruction is removed.

## MYTHS AND MISCONCEPTIONS

"Slap the choking victim
on her back."

### JUST THE FACTS:

During a choking incident, the windpipe structure goes into spasm to prevent the foreign object from moving down into the lungs. Banging the victim on the back usually will not dislodge the obstruction. What will help is causing the air trapped in the lungs to be expelled quickly, causing the object in the air passage to pop out. This can be accomplished by pushing up on the diaphragm into the lungs with abdominal thrusts.

## Special Choking Situations

If the choking person is a pregnant woman or rotund person, do a chest thrust. Place your fist and hand over lower half of victim's breastbone. Repeatedly pull/thrust straight back until object is dislodged. If victim is taller than you, have him kneel down first, then position yourself.

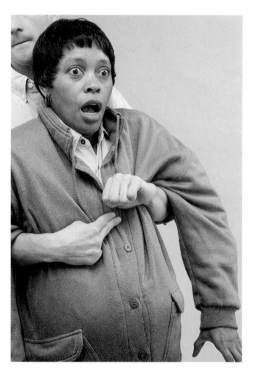

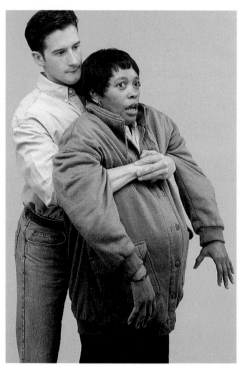

Infants and toddlers are especially vulnerable to choking because of their habit of putting everything in their mouths. Their immature airway structure also puts them at greater risk of choking.

In general, life support procedures for a choking child (ages 1–8) are very similar to those of an adult—just don't squeeze as hard. You may also need to position yourself on your knees to get to their level.

Infants and most young toddlers (under 12–18 months) must be treated differently.

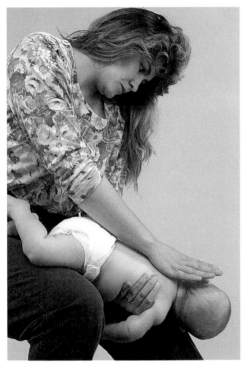

Hold the infant face down on your forearm. Be sure to support the head and neck.

Deliver five back blows forcefully between the shoulder blades. Use the heel of your hand.

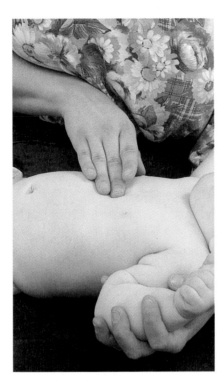

Turn infant face up on your arm. Be sure to support the infant's head. Using two fingers, provide five downward chest thrusts on the breastbone, one finger width below an imaginary line drawn between the nipples.

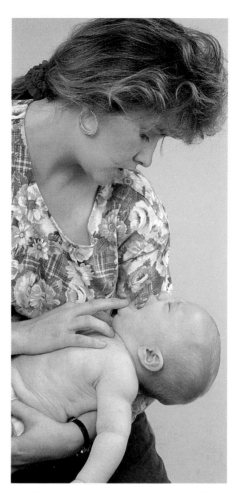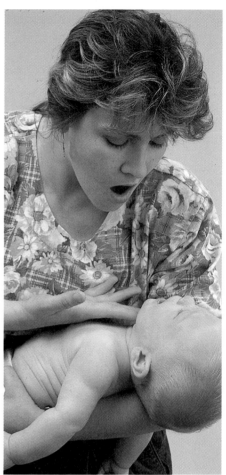

Look in the mouth and remove the foreign object only if you can see it.

Open the airway and attempt rescue breathing. If the chest does not rise, reposition the airway and try again.

If the airway remains blocked, repeat back blows and chest thrusts, and attempt to breathe for the infant until the object is removed and ventilations are successful.

# If You Are Alone and Choke

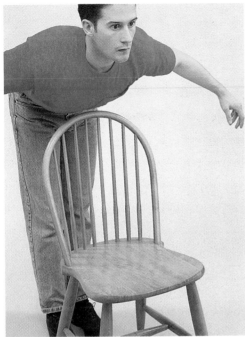

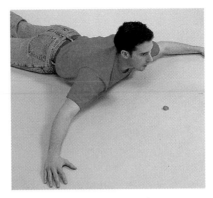

Throw yourself to the floor to "knock the wind out" of yourself.

Forcefully propel yourself over a chair or other firm object.

## DON'T LET IT HAPPEN TO YOU

The usual causes of choking in adults are easy to **C**.

> CUTTING FOOD INTO PIECES THAT ARE TOO LARGE.
> CHEWING FOOD IMPROPERLY (ESPECIALLY WITH DENTURES).
> CHATTING AND TALKING WITH FOOD IN YOUR MOUTH (ESPECIALLY WHEN YOUR NOSE IS CONGESTED FROM A COLD OR ALLERGY).
> COCKTAILS—DRINKING TOO MUCH ALCOHOL WHILE EATING CAN AFFECT SWALLOWING AND/OR GAG REFLEX.

## SUPPORT AIRWAY SUMMARY

- ❏ **Observe for problems**
- ❏ **Chin lift**
- ❏ **Clear the mouth**
- ❏ **Body position**
- ❏ **Jaw thrust**
- ❏ **Heimlich maneuver**

*You can do it!*

# CHAPTER 5

## SUPPORT BREATHING

That a patient is breathing on his own is a good sign, but the ill or injured person can still use your help to make his breathing process as effective as possible. You can help to insure continued maximum amount of oxygen to the brain (i.e., "Juice to the squash").

It is important to continue to observe the breathing by looking, listening, and feeling for the exchange of air.

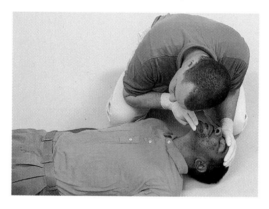

The next supportive action is to keep the victim of suspected serious illness or injury in the position that will help make the working of the lungs as efficient as possible. For most patients the BEST POSITION is flat on the back.

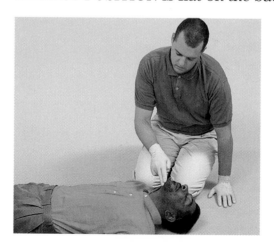

If a conscious patient complains of difficulty breathing or discomfort lying flat, allow him to sit up or assume the position most comfortable for him.

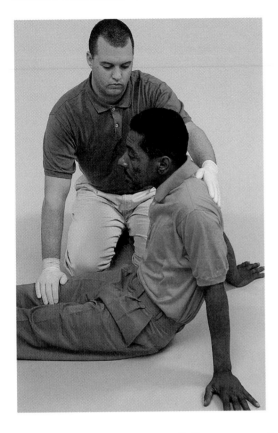

Open windows and doors to enhance the availability of ambient oxygen. Attempt to keep needless bystanders and onlookers away from the area (i.e., crowd control).

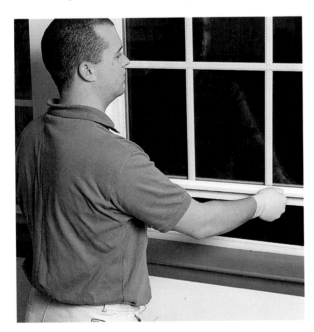

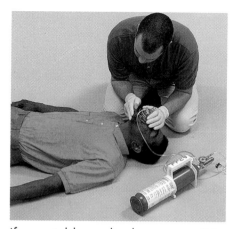

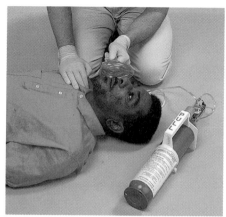

If a portable medical oxygen unit is available, provide the patient with this supplemental oxygen as soon as possible. Continue to maintain airway and to closely monitor continued breathing when oxygen is being administered.

If a conscious patient resists you placing an oxygen mask over his face, simply hold the oxygen mask *near* his face.

Be careful to observe for vomiting or secretions that could cause an airway obstruction.

## HELPFUL BACKGROUND INFORMATION

"Room air" normally contains about 21 percent oxygen. The average person uses only about one quarter of that oxygen with each breath for normal brain and body function. When a person is suddenly ill or injured, a more concentrated source of oxygen will improve the efficiency of breathing and help slow down the "shutdown" process.

Because oxygen units vary in function and complexity, it is important to follow the manufacturer's instructions for use, maintenance and service. Typical oxygen devices may provide either fixed flow (i.e., a predetermined flow rate) or variable flow (a range of flow rates). For emergency use, a minimum flow of six liters per minute is required. Emergency oxygen units are available as nonprescription devices either by direct purchase or by leasing from oxygen service companies.

If you have a medical oxygen unit at your location, it should be kept where it is easily accessible. Oxygen units should be portable and simple to operate (the simpler the better). Your familiarity with the device will improve the efficiency of your emergency response; practice using it and inspect it regularly to be sure it is full.

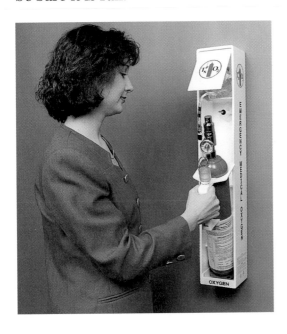

## SUPPORT BREATHING SUMMARY

❏ **Look, listen, and feel for breathing**
❏ **Find best position for ease of breathing**
❏ **Improve fresh air quantity (if possible)**
❏ **Give medical oxygen as soon as available**
❏ **Keep onlookers away**

# You can do it!

# CHAPTER 6

## SUPPORT CIRCULATION

Supporting circulation involves actions to insure that the heart, blood vessels, and blood can supply oxygen to the brain and other vital body tissues as best they can under the circumstances.

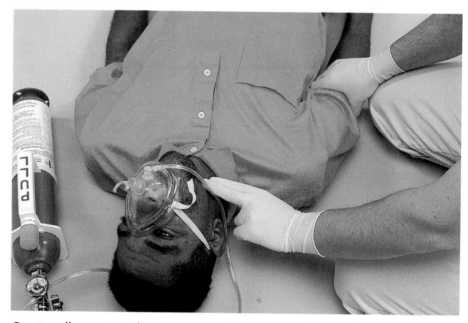

Continually monitor the presence of heart action by gently feeling the neck for a pulse.

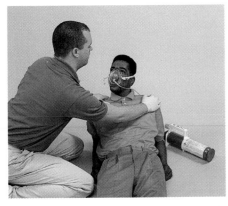

Minimize the body's need for blood supply by keeping the ill or injured person at rest.

Often denial and emotions may result in the patient wanting to move about. Don't let him do so.

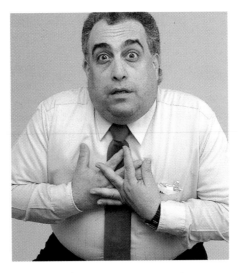

Keeping the patient at complete rest takes on special importance when he is experiencing chest pain or other indications of a possible heart attack or other heart-related problems.

## Helpful Background Information

Simply described, a heart attack occurs when one or more of the major arteries serving the heart becomes blocked or narrows to a point whereby blood cannot reach a portion of the heart muscle. The area of the heart wall thus deprived of oxygenated blood will die. While other parts of the heart muscle will attempt to continue to function, the resulting complications can be catastrophic and can result in sudden death.

Outside of a sophisticated medical service it is virtually impossible to deal with the chemical, electrical, and/or physical complications that can follow a heart attack. However, early recognition of warning signs, a prompt call for medical help, and initial life support actions can minimize the occurrence of these complications.

Early warning signs of a possible heart attack:

- Chest pain, pressure, discomfort, or tightness (lasting more than two minutes)
- Pain in left arm, neck, jaw, or back
- Weakness, lightheadedness, or anxiety
- Nausea and/or sweating
- Denial that anything is wrong

## POSSIBLE HEART PROBLEMS

A person with these symptoms may be having a heart attack. But it could also be a far less serious problem (for example, indigestion, stress, or a hiatal hernia). It is difficult to know for sure. It's much better to go to the hospital, find out it's not serious, and be embarrassed than to ignore the symptoms and be dead!

The sooner a possible heart attack victim receives advanced cardiac care, the more likely modern medicine can help avert the chemical, electrical, and physical complications that can and do kill heart attack patients.

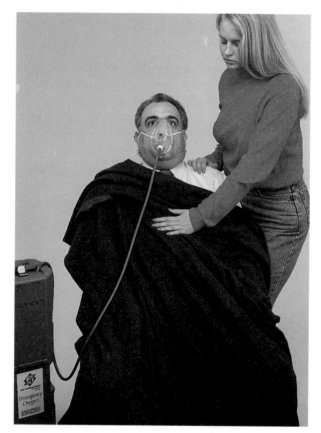

If someone is having any combination of these signs and symptoms, immediately call for medical help and initiate ABCS life support measures.

Keep the patient in a comfortable position, reassure him, and improve air quality and/or administer oxygen.

## DON'T LET IT HAPPEN TO YOU

Heart disease continues to be the number one cause of death. Although early detection and rapid intervention are crucial to treating heart problems, prevention is the only sure way to decrease premature cardiac death.

Modern medical science has determined a number of factors that increase the risk of heart attacks. Some of these common factors, such as age, gender, and family history, cannot be changed. However, the collective behaviors known as Healthy Heart Actions can have a dramatic effect on reducing the likelihood and onset of heart disease. To insure a healthy heart:

- Eat well (low fat).
- Exercise regularly (3–5 times a week).
- Recognize and limit the effects of stress.
- Get enough and proper sleep.

If necessary,

- Take prescribed medications (especially for heart problems or high blood pressure).
- Control diabetes.

The most important of all Healthy Heart Actions . . .

- Be SMOKE FREE!

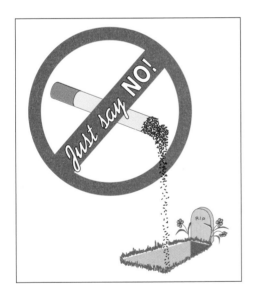

## CONTROL ALL SERIOUS BLEEDING

Helping the heart to be as efficient as possible is only part of supporting circulation. You will also need to control any serious external bleeding. The average adult body contains 12 pints of blood. Loss of more than one pint results in loss of a significant number of oxygen-carrying red blood cells and can also result in dangerous lowering of blood pressure. Serious bleeding usually will not stop by itself; you have to help.

## MYTHS AND MISCONCEPTIONS

"Touching or coming into contact with someone who is bleeding can cause AIDS or Hepatitis."

**JUST THE FACTS:**

The mere sight of blood is repulsive to many people. Now there is the added fear of diseases that can be transmitted via blood or other body fluids from one person to another.

The fear of contracting a so-called blood-borne pathogen through contact with a patient's external bleeding is far greater than the actual threat. Nevertheless, the serious consequences of HIV (the virus that causes AIDS) or HBV (the hepatitis virus that causes serious liver damage) warrant precautions when dealing with bleeding from a stranger or someone with whom you are not intimate.

AIDS is nearly always a fatal disease. The AIDS epidemic has achieved alarming proportions and has reached into every segment of our society—rich or poor, gay or straight, black, white, or yellow—so that no one person or group practicing risky behavior is safe from infection.

The best scientific data indicates that to be transmitted from one person to another, the HIV virus has to be present in sufficient concentration in one of three body fluids: blood, semen, or vaginal secretions (or other body fluids containing one of these three fluids). The contaminated fluid then has to enter the body of a noninfected person.

There are only three documented modes of transmission of the HIV virus: sexual conduct, blood to blood, or from a mother to her baby during pregnancy or at birth.

## DON'T LET IT HAPPEN TO YOU

In greatest danger are those who practice risky social behaviors. Nearly 90% of all AIDS victims are those who engaged in unprotected sex with multiple partners or who shared IV needles. (It must be noted, however, that HIV can be transmitted in just one sex act or one episode of needle sharing.)

Although health care workers and emergency medical responders are believed to be at high risk, remarkably few have been infected. The reasons are clear: Health care workers reduce their risk by following reasonable precautions in their work.

Because AIDS is so often fatal, and because medical science and society still don't know everything there is to know about the dreaded disease, direct contact with the blood or body fluids of a potentially infected person during a medical emergency should be avoided.

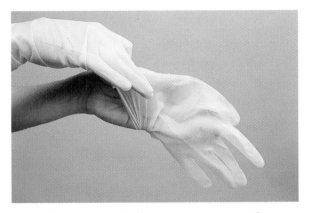

To reduce your risk of contacting or catching a blood-borne disease during a medical emergency, wear latex gloves.

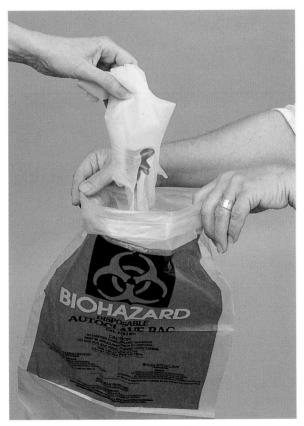

Properly dispose of all materials soiled by blood or body secretions in a watertight waste container clearly labeled "Biohazard Waste."

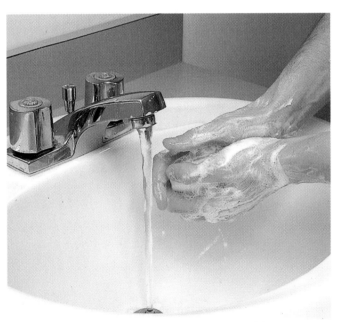

Don't forget to wash your hands thoroughly as soon as convenient to do so.

# Controlling Bleeding

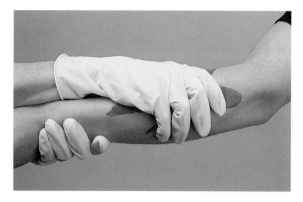

The best method to control serious bleeding is direct pressure. To accomplish this, place a gauze dressing or other clean cloth over the bleeding site and press firmly with your hand.

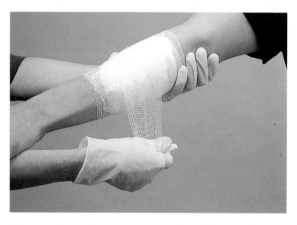

Using a bandaging material such as roller gauze, apply and secure the dressing material in place with firm pressure.

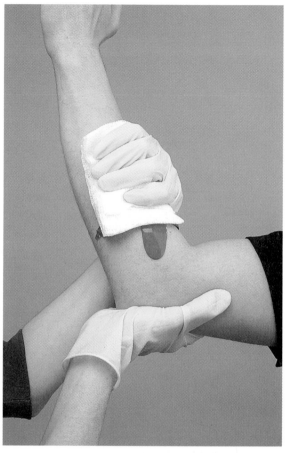

Elevate the bleeding site **if possible**, i.e., to do so will not cause additional harm to the limb.

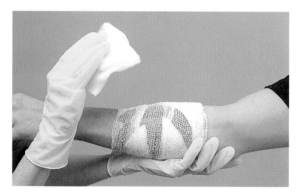

If bleeding continues through the bandage, add more dressing over the initial bandage.

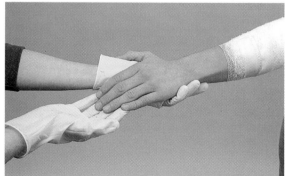

If at all possible, leave fingers and toes exposed so you can check for adequate circulation.

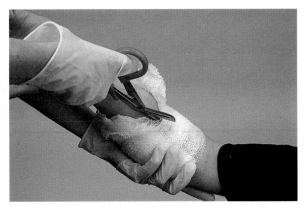

If fingers and toes become discolored, numb, or feel cold, loosen the bandage, preferably by cutting it. Afterward, simply apply more bandaging material over the initial material.

## HELPFUL BACKGROUND INFORMATION

Clotting is a natural body defense process and the only way that bleeding ultimately will be stopped. Clotting occurs when certain components in the blood (platelets) mix with air and congeal. That is why it's important to use a porous dressing material that will allow air to pass through. Using an occlusive material that keeps air out will hinder the clotting process.

In effect, applying direct pressure and/or a pressure bandage will assist the body's own natural defense mechanism. Blood will not clot when it is pouring out. Your actions will help clotting occur. Bandaging a serious bleeding wound is neither an art form nor a science—it simply has to do the job. Try to use clean, fine-meshed material directly on the wound for dressing and bandages.

Do not apply the bandage too loosely. This will allow a dressing to slip and will put no pressure on the wound. However, be careful not to apply the bandage too tightly. A bandage must be snug enough to hold a dressing in place and exert pressure on the wound, but it must not be so tight that it will interfere with circulation.

### IMPORTANT POINT

A dressing should never be removed until the wound is being cleaned and/or medically treated (e.g., sutured). You risk dislodging clots and causing more bleeding if you remove a dressing too soon.

### IMPORTANT POINT

Avoid towels and other such absorbent materials. Remember, you want to help control the bleeding, not collect it.

## MYTHS AND MISCONCEPTIONS

"Use a tourniquet or pressure
points to stop external bleeding."

**JUST THE FACTS:**

A tourniquet may well stop external bleeding from an extremity, but there is a very real danger of doing further damage to the limb. A properly applied tourniquet will stop the flow of blood from a wound, but it can also interrupt the flow of blood to the cells and tissue of the injured extremity, frequently resulting in needless amputation. In other words, why stop the bleeding at the risk of structural damage?

Releasing and reapplying the tourniquet every few minutes is not a solution to these problems because toxins accumulated at the wound site could be absorbed into the body and cause a serious case of toxic shock. Only after all else fails or when there is no time for direct pressure (as may be the case when there are multiple victims) should a tourniquet be considered.

"Pressure points" have been taught as a bleeding control procedure for years. However, there is little clinical evidence that they actually work well and they are difficult to remember and find. Moreover, applying digital pressure at pulse points is time consuming and can take you away from dealing with airway and breathing problems.

## ENHANCE BLOOD VOLUME

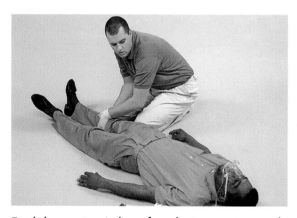

Feel the patient's legs for obvious pain, tenderness, or deformity.

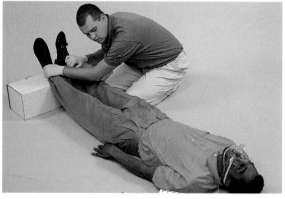

If possible, raise the patient's legs 12–18 inches to provide additional oxygen-carrying red blood cells to the heart, lungs, and brain.

## Maintain Body Temperature

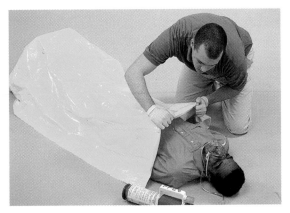

You can further support the working of the heart, vessels, and blood by covering any ill or injured person with a blanket or some such material.

## EXCEPTION

Do not raise the legs if they appear to be injured or if there is an obvious head injury. In the case of a head injury, raising the legs will increase "juice to the squash" but may do additional harm by increasing the amount of fluid around the brain.

## HELPFUL BACKGROUND INFORMATION

One of the effects of shock is a shutdown in the body's heat regulation system. As patients lose body heat they become hypothermic (a lowering of the body temperature). During hypothermia the musculature of the heart and blood vessels sustains greatly reduced effectiveness, thus worsening an already compromised cardiovascular system.

A blanket or other such cover is not intended to warm up a victim, but rather will reflect lost body heat back into the patient. In most situations, covering a sick or injured person with one blanket and tucking it around him will be sufficient to maintain body heat. If, however, the surface on which the person is lying is very cold, a blanket placed under him will help insulate and prevent body heat from transferring into the cold surface.

## CAUTION

If you suspect the patient has a spinal injury, DO NOT move him to place a blanket under him.

## SUPPORT CIRCULATION SUMMARY

❑ **Check the pulse.**

❑ **Keep patient at complete rest.**

❑ **Control external bleeding.**

❑ **Elevate uninjured legs.**

❑ **Cover with a blanket or coat.**

## *You can do it!*

# CHAPTER 7

## SUPPORT SPINE

Supporting the function of the spine and minimizing the likelihood of a spinal cord injury is an important life support function in all victims suspected of sustaining a mechanism of injury such as a fall, auto accident, diving into shallow water, or sledding accident.

Heart and lung action are both triggered by signals from the brain. Interruption of these signals, caused by a severed spinal cord or from pressure on the cord, can result in sudden death with no hope of resuscitation. In addition, damage to the spinal cord or mishandling of the victim after the accident can result in a victim being permanently crippled if he survives. There is not much you can do to help an already damaged spinal cord, but there is a lot you can do to limit the complications of a damaged spinal column.

### IMMOBILIZE HEAD AND NECK

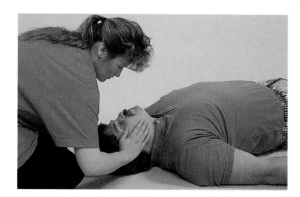

If your Quik Chek findings indicate a possible spine injury, keep the victim from moving. Immobilize the head and neck by cradling the head with both of your hands. If the patient is unconscious, utilize the jaw thrust to maintain the airway from this position.

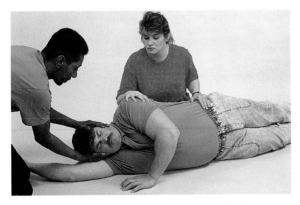

If movement becomes necessary to help maintain airway and breathing, carefully "log roll" the patient by moving his body as a unit.

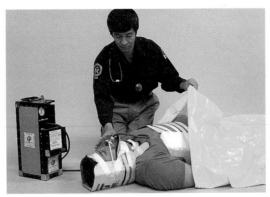

EMS professionals and others trained to do so, will usually place a rigid cervical collar on the patient and place him on a spinal immobilization device before transporting or relocating him.

## DON'T LET IT HAPPEN TO YOU

The primary causes of head and neck injuries are slips and falls (at work or at home) and auto accidents on the road. In highway mishaps, properly worn safety belts significantly reduce the likelihood of serious skull and/or spinal injury. Even on short trips around the neighborhood, always wear your safety belt (80 percent of auto accidents occur less than 25 miles from home).

Slips and falls usually result from wet floors or wearing inadequate footwear for a specific task or job. clean up all spills immediately. Even water can cause someone to lose his footing. Always wear appropriate shoes or boots for a particular environment or activity.

Unfortunately, regardless of seat belts and footwear, a major factor in many injuries is inappropriate use of alcohol. Never drink then drive or work. Various regulations have allowable blood alcohol concentration (BAC) levels, but remember: BAC is a limit, not a goal. The best BAC for driving and working is 0.0!

If you do choose to use alcohol at appropriate times and places, keep in mind that it will affect your coordination. Moreover, exceeding your personal pleasure level when drinking alcohol will result in some degree of a hangover. Most people would never drink at work or go to work intoxicated. However, hangovers will also decrease perception, alertness, and reflexes, which can result in dangerous slips and falls at home or at work.

## SUPPORT SPINE SUMMARY

❑ Based on mechanism of injury/survey findings.

❑ Manually immobilize head.

❑ Don't move patient or parts.

❑ Log roll if movement is absolutely necessary.

## You can do it!

# FIRST CARE CHEKSHEET™

## "QUIK CHEK"™

✓ **Check The Area**
- ☐ Hazards
- ☐ Latex Gloves

✓ **Do No Harm**
- ☐ Responsiveness?

✓ **Call Out for Help**
- ☐ Body Position

**A –Airway**
- ☐ Chin Position
- ☐ Obstruction

**B –Breathing**
- ☐ Look
- ☐ Listen
- ☐ Feel

✓ **Seek Medical Help???**

**C –Circulation**
- ☐ Pulse
- ☐ Bleeding

**S –Spine**
- ☐ Mechanism of Injury
- ☐ Neck
- ☐ Head
- ☐ Limb Sensation

✓ **Support Life**

✓ **Make the Right Call (EMS)???**

## ✓ Support Life

**A** ☐ Airway Maintained
- ☐ Mouth Cleared
- ☐ Heimlich Maneuver
- ☐ Positioned on Side **???**
- ☐ Jaw Thrust **???**

**B** ☐ Breathing Watched
- ☐ Oxygen
- ☐ Best Position _____
- ☐ Fresh Air
- ☐ Crowd Control

**C** ☐ Pulse Checked
- ☐ Complete Rest
- ☐ Controlled Bleeding
  Where _____
  How _____
- ☐ Burns Cooled/Covered
- ☐ Legs Elevated **???**
- ☐ Cover/Blanket

**S** ☐ Don't Move Patient/Parts
- ☐ Log Roll **???**
- ☐ Immobilize Head

## *You can do it!*

# CHAPTER 8

# SPECIFIC ILLNESS AND INJURY SITUATIONS

ABCS CARE is the basic response plan for all potentially serious medical emergencies in which the patient is breathing and has a pulse. As we introduced you to the ABCS CARE plan, we presented a few specific problems and/or exceptional situations (i.e. heart attacks, seizures, face trauma, etc.) In this unit we will present the application of the Emergency First Care in several other specific illness and injury situations.

No matter what the medical emergency may be, your basic plan remains the same:

1. Check The area
   - Neutralize hazards/wear latex gloves
2. Do No Harm
   - Don't move body or parts (unnecessarily)
3. Send or call for help
   - MAKE THE RIGHT CALL (EMS)
4. Support Life
   - ABCS—Check 'em and make 'em the best they can be!

## AMPUTATION

A person's extremity or a portion of an extremity severed from the body is a gruesome sight. However, don't be distracted by or focus on the amputated part. Unless it is a decapitation (in which case there's nothing anyone can do), people don't usually die from the amputation of a body part. They die from the complications to **a**irway, **b**reathing, **c**irculation, and **s**pine. Stick to your plan and your priorities, as listed above.

# Additional Actions (if necessary and possible)

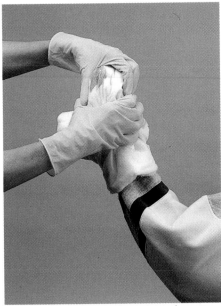

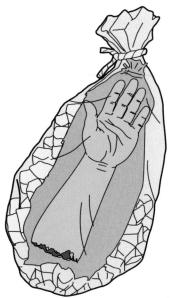

Apply direct pressure over the site of amputation.

Elevate the limb or "stump" as long as to do so will not cause additional harm to the limb. Note: Because of the elasticity of major blood vessels, which "snap up" and close off when severed, there may very well be little or no bleeding at the amputation site.

After you have supported the patient's ABCS, care for the amputated part.
- Find it.
- Wrap it in something clean.
- Keep it dry (a plastic bag or bowl will help).
- Keep it cool.
- Transport part with patient to medical facility.
- Continue to check and support patient's ABCS!

## CAUTION

**Place it *on* ice but don't place it *in* ice and risk freezing or frostbite of the severed part.**

## HELPFUL BACKGROUND INFORMATION

If you support life in the person who has sustained a traumatic amputation, you have helped to insure his survival and helped make it possible for medical professionals to do their job. If the patient survives, the miracle of modern microsurgery can often reattach severed limbs and/or digits.

There have been successful reattachments up to eight to ten hours after the accident. These repaired extremities don't always have the full abilities present before the accident, but they are often better than artificial limbs, both psychologically and physiologically.

# BURNS

Burn wounds present a unique problem for First Care Givers. While they are perhaps the easiest of all wounds to care for, they often present an emotional challenge that could hinder proper response to the situation.

The mere thought of burns or burning frightens us. We learned as very young toddlers, "Don't touch the stove!" "Don't play with matches!" "Don't go near the radiator!" Many of us have learned "hands on" that hot hurts!

At the time of a burn emergency the patient is often in tremendous pain and very frightened. The sights and/or smells of burned human flesh tend to be very disturbing to the victim *and* First Care Giver alike. Your emotional reactions are normal, but you must not let your emotions prevent you from helping the patient.

## MYTHS AND MISCONCEPTIONS

Determine the degree of burn
and percent of body burned.

### JUST THE FACTS:

In medical centers, burns are defined by the depth of tissue involvement (usually as first, second, or third degree) and the percent of the body burned. But for the First Care Giver it doesn't matter what the degree of burn is or how much of the body surface is affected. Your Emergency First Care actions are the same for all burn patients.

## Actions for Burns from Fire/Heat

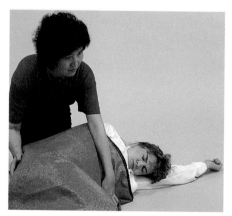

Stop all burning and/or remove source of heat. (If patient is still burning, stop him, drop him, roll him or cover with a blanket.)

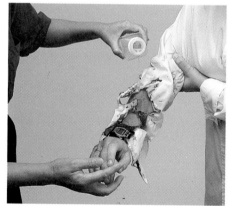

Stop the burning process with cool water or other nontoxic liquid.

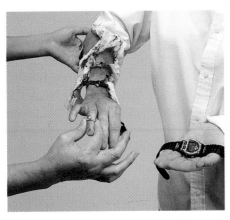

Remove jewelry (if any) in affected area.

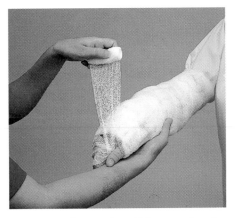

For minor (superficial) burns: Apply dry dressing and bandage.

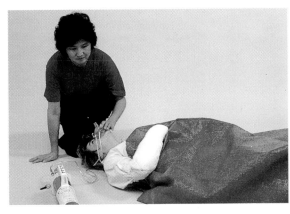

For serious burn injury:
- Apply cool water only until the burning has stopped.
- Administer oxygen.
- Cover the burned area with dry dressing, sheet, or cleanest available material.
- Cover person to prevent loss of body heat.
- Closely monitor ABCS. (Be sure to give oxygen if available.)
- Get medical help.

## Actions for Chemical Burns

Remove all affected clothing as you flush the area with large amounts of water for at least thirty (30) minutes. (Burns from powdered chemicals should be brushed or blown off before flushing with water.) Provide ABCS CARE. Call for medical help/transport.

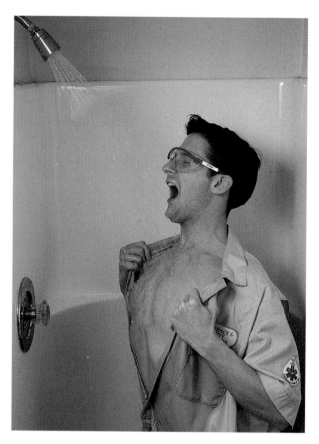

### Chemical in Eyes

Immediately flush eye with water or clear liquid for about 15 minutes. (If available, an eye-wash station is well designed for this.) If only one eye is involved, wash from bridge of nose out. (Try to avoid contamination of the unaffected eye.) You may have to hold eyelids open gently during irrigation. After irrigation, cover eye with moist dressing. Provide ABCS CARE and seek medical attention.

## Electrical Burns

Turn off the power or safely remove the source of electricity from the patient. Do a Quik Chek and give ABCS CARE. Do CPR if necessary. Locate and cover entrance and exit wounds. Closely watch and support ABCS. Call for medical help.

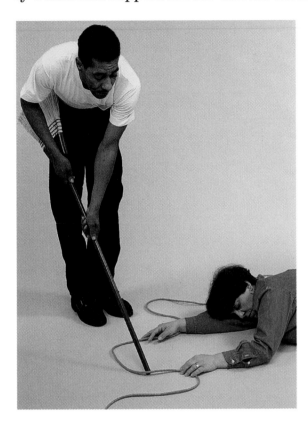

## IMPALED OBJECT

Should you find someone with a knife, arrow, rod, pole, or anything else protruding from his body, DO NOT PULL IT OUT. The object may well be acting like a cork. Removal may result in serious bleeding or additional internal damage. Your priorities and Emergency First Care plan of action remain the same:

1. Check The Area

2. Do No Harm

3. Get Help

4. Support Life: Provide ABCS CARE

## Additional Actions

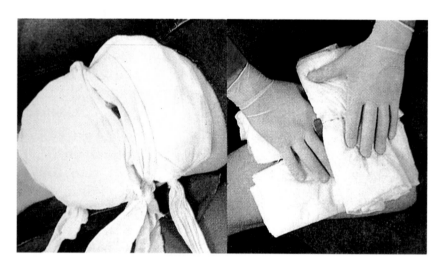

After you support life, secure the object and pad around it if possible to control any bleeding and prevent the object from becoming dislodged. Continue to check and support patient's ABCS.

## Exception: Object in Face

If someone has an object impaled in his cheek and the object has entered the mouth cavity, gently remove it. The possibility of blood blocking the airway is an even greater threat. Attempt to control the bleeding by applying pressure from both inside and outside the cheek. Place the victim on his side to allow for drainage.

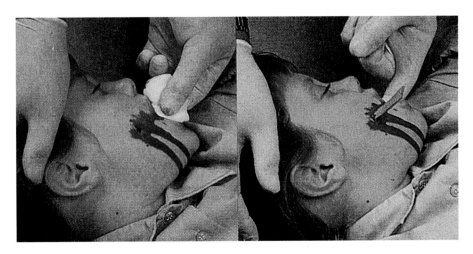

### Object in Eye

Secure impaled object from further movement using a cup or something similar. Cover good eye to prevent sympathetic eye movement of injured eye.

   Provide emotional support and encouragement to patient. Keep checking and supporting ABCS! Seek medical attention.

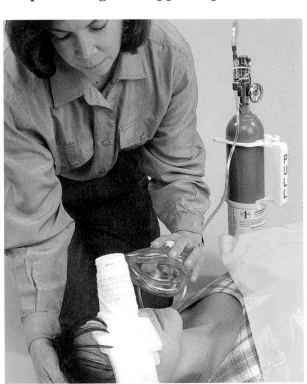

**IMPORTANT POINT**

**DO NOT REMOVE AN OBJECT STUCK IN EYE!**

## POISONING

A poison is any toxic substance which can negatively affect mental or breathing function in living creatures. Poisoning in humans generally occurs via skin contact, injestion, injection, or inhalation.

Someone can become a victim of poisoning from chemicals (liquid or vapors), drugs (legal or illegal), or venom (bites or stings).

Most poisonings, especially in children, are accidental; but sadly some teenagers and adults sometimes use poison to end their lives.

### Additional Actions

After assuring your own safety and initiating ABCS CARE, call the Poison Control Center or EMS in your community. (At a worksite, you should also refer to available MSDS sheets for the chemical(s) involved.) Depending on the situation and if possible, be prepared to provide the following information:

- Type of poison, chemical or drug.
- Method of contact (injestion, injection, or inhalation).
- Estimated amount of poison or type of insect/snake.
- Age and size of victim.
- Victim's condition (especially mental and breathing status).

Poison Control Center (or EMS dispatcher) instructions may include giving fluids or an antidote or inducing vomiting. Follow advice given as best you can and continue to provide ABCS CARE until help arrives or you transport the victim to medical care.

**CAUTION**

If inhalation is suspected, shut off source of gas or vapors before entering the area or wear proper respirator and/or apparel to protect yourself. A "one-way" valve may be necessary for CPR.

**CAUTION**

Never give fluids to or induce vomiting in a victim who isn't totally conscious.

# PART 3

## CARE UNTIL PROFESSIONAL MEDICAL HELP IS AVAILABLE

Although the priorities of Emergency First Care are Airway, Breathing, Circulation, and Spine, **CARE** for the victim of sudden illness or serious injury is also essential and must be delivered as life support is provided.

The dictionary defines *care* as "serious attention, watchfulness, to feel interest in, to be concerned." These definitions also well describe the Emergency First Care acronym **CARE**. As life-sustaining ABCS are supported, the First Care Giver must also:

COMMUNICATE
AVOID HARM
REEXAMINE
ENCOURAGE

# CHAPTER 9

## COMMUNICATE

Communication is an ongoing and essential part of Emergency First Care. Your ability to communicate effectively with the patient, medical services, and others possibly involved in an emergency medical situation may have significant impact on the outcome.

## IMPORTANT POINT

Even if there is no response from the patient, talk to him. Hearing is the last sense to leave the body and the first to return after sleep or unconsciousness. (How often do you lie in bed in the morning waiting for your alarm clock to go off? Yet you *hear* it!) Seemingly unconscious people often hear and react emotionally to things said around them.

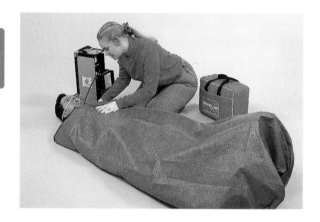

## TALK TO PATIENT

As you provide ABC'S Life Support, be sure to talk to the ill or injured person. Every time you touch him or do something for him, let them know what you are going to do.

Tell the victim your name. Even if he knew you before the event, intense emotions or lack of oxygen to the brain could leave him confused.

Tell him that you have had First Care training, ask if you can help, and inform him that professional medical help is on the way.

## NOTIFY APPROPRIATE PEOPLE

If you are at work, alert your Medical Response Team, involve co-workers in helping you, and as soon as possible inform your supervisor or manager about the incident.

Know your workplace emergency response plan and how to summon help. Worksite emergency numbers and/or procedures for contacting medical advice services should be posted at every telephone or two-way radio.

## MAKE THE RIGHT CALL (EMS)

When your Keen Sense of the Obvious (KSO) indicates that someone is experiencing a possible life-threatening episode, call for EMS services as soon as possible. If you're at home, summon and involve other family members or nearby neighbors.

In many communities the numbers to dial on your telephone are 911. If your community doesn't use this emergency number, have your local number posted at all phones in your home or workplace.

Deciding to call for help and actually placing the call are often very emotional experiences. Those emotional energies can be effectively channeled by having an Emergency Action Plan to follow.

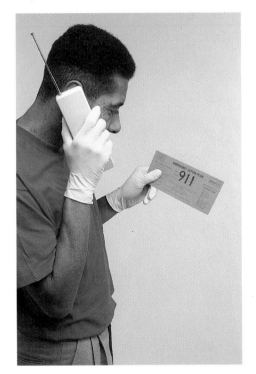

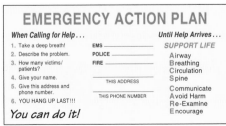

Emergency Action Plan card

## WRITE IT DOWN!

Recording your findings and actions at the time of a medical emergency can provide you with a useful tool for passing information along to the medical people.

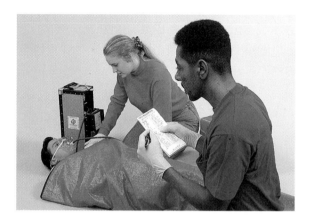

Making a brief written record at the time of the emergency will also assist you in completing more detailed forms and reports that may be required by your employer after the emergency. If you write it down, you are more likely to remember it.

As you do a Quik Chek and ABCS CARE, it's ok if you or someone with you uses a checklist to be sure you don't overlook anything important.

An easy access checklist also gives you a logical point of reference for talking to and communicating with EMS and other medical professionals when they take over care of the patient.

## COMMUNICATE SUMMARY

❑ **Talk to the patient.**

❑ **Seek medical help.**

❑ **Inform appropriate people.**

❑ **Record findings and care given.**

## *You can do it!*

# CHAPTER 10

## AVOID HARM

As prescribed by Golden Rule #2, do not cause more harm to the patient. This unit describes some additional concerns and cautions as you support life and wait for medical professionals to arrive.

The goal of Emergency First Care is not only to minimize but also to avoid causing physical complications in an emergency patient. Don't make the situation worse by your actions.

## NO FOOD OR DRINK

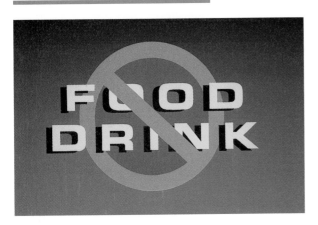

Although it may not seem the compassionate thing to do, don't allow a seriously ill or injured person anything to ingest. Anything swallowed could be vomited, which could cause three complications:

1. The airway could become blocked by solid vomit.

2. The vomited secretions could be drawn into the lungs, resulting in serious breathing difficulties.

3. It's not very pleasant to get it on you or clean it up.

**NEVER PUT ANY-THING LIQUID OR SOLID INTO THE MOUTH OF AN UNCONSCIOUS PERSON.**

## Possible Exception

If you know that an ill person is a diabetic and he appears to be weak, irritable, and/or confused (with no other major obvious problems), consider giving her some sugar in the form of a sweetened soft drink or other beverage.

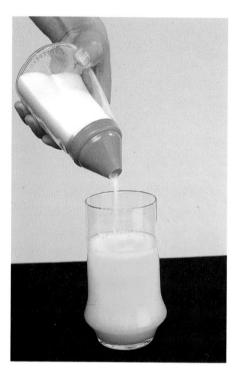
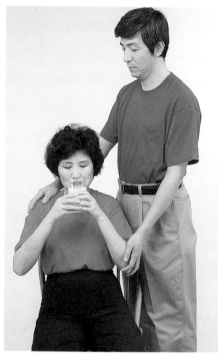

Give a sweetened beverage to such a patient only if:

- They can hold it!
- They can drink it without your help.

### MYTHS AND MISCONCEPTIONS

"Place some sugar around the lips and gums of an unconscious diabetic."

**JUST THE FACTS:**
It is highly unlikely that solid sugar or even commercially available sugar paste will be adequately absorbed by an unconscious patient in a diabetic crisis. Moreover, anything in the mouth of an unconscious patient can cause a serious airway problem.

## HELPFUL BACKGROUND INFORMATION

The body and brain cells not only require oxygen for survival, they also need sugar. Most food consumed is converted into various forms of sugar during digestion. This sugar is absorbed and carried by blood throughout the body.

In order for this sugar in the blood to pass into the cells, it must be aided by a chemical substance known as insulin.

A diabetic is a person whose pancreas is not producing sufficient insulin. Diabetics can still lead normal lives by carefully controlling their food intake and periodically taking artificial insulin.

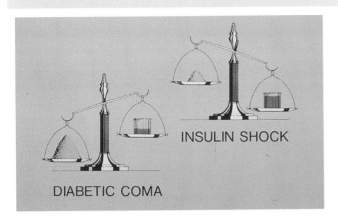

INSULIN SHOCK

DIABETIC COMA

This balance between food (converted to sugar) and artificial insulin is very delicate. Too much insulin or not enough sugar will result in significant "shut down" problems in the brain of a diabetic. Whether the patient is suffering diabetic coma (too much sugar, not enough insulin) or insulin shock (too much insulin, not enough sugar) is difficult for the First Care Giver to determine immediately.

Fortunately, you don't need to differentiate between the two; ABCS CARE actions are the same for both. In addition, all conscious diabetic emergency patients should receive a sweet drink. The insulin shock patient will usually show dramatic improvement.

If a known diabetic shows no immediate improvement, immediate medical care must be sought.

## CAUTION

Never give insulin to a suddenly ill diabetic.

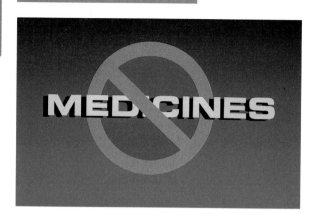

# GIVE NO MEDICINE

Pills and potions are not the answer to all medical problems, especially emergency situations. Unless it is specifically ordered by a physician, don't give an ill or injured person any drugs or medication.

## HELPFUL BACKGROUND INFORMATION

Nitroglycerin is a vasodilator. Its action in the body is to temporarily widen the coronary arteries to allow more blood to reach a heart muscle experiencing pain or discomfort due to coronary artery blockage or spasm. But it doesn't affect only coronary arteries, it opens many blood vessels in the body. This can significantly lower blood pressure and result in an inability to deliver oxygen to the brain (big-time shutdown!).

Nitroglycerin comes in tiny white pills and is stored in small brown bottles.

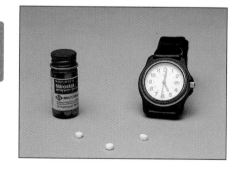

## Administering Nitroglycerin

When helping someone who is having chest pain or discomfort to take their own prescription of nitroglycerin:

1. Be sure the patient is awake.
2. Place one tiny white pill under the tongue (it will dissolve there).
3. If there is no relief from the discomfort within five minutes, place a second pill under their tongue.
4. If no relief within another five minutes, give a third pill.
5. Then put the medicine away and, if no relief, get medical help.

   Expect that the patient will complain of a headache after taking nitroglycerin.

## AVOID ROUGH HANDLING

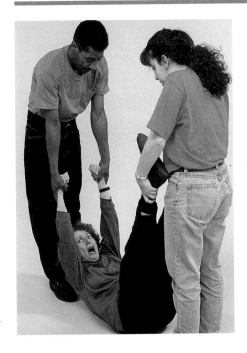

Be gentle when touching or doing something to an emergency patient. Causing more pain can make shock worse and can also affect the patient's confidence and trust in your ability to help her.

## POSSIBLE FRACTURE, SPRAIN, OR DISLOCATION

Don't move suspected limb injuries. If you see or hear the patient complaining of . . .

- pain or tenderness
- swelling
- deformity

- discoloration (at the injury site)

. . . there is a POSSIBILITY that a broken bone or serious joint injury exists. Whether or not it is broken, sprained, or strained, gently and carefully IMMOBILIZE the part by "splinting it where it lies."

The decision to splint an extremity injury and what device or material to use depends on the presence of other more serious problems, how soon medical help will arrive, and what you have available to use.

If better-trained and -equipped help is minutes away (and the victim is not in an immediate hazard or danger), the best splint is the ground, floor, or deck (think about it—it's always there and always the right size). LEAVE HER WHERE SHE IS AND DON'T MOVE THE BODY OR ITS PARTS.

The second-best splint is the body of the injured person. If necessary you may be able to splint an injured area directly to the body.

## REMEMBER

The priority for a person with a limb injury is still life support for the ABCS.

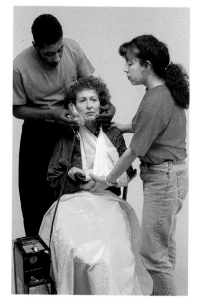
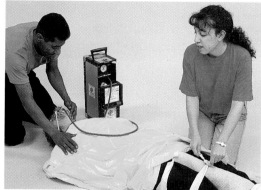

## SUMMARY OF AVOID HARM

❑ **No food or drink.**
❑ **No medicine (unless ordered by physician).**
❑ **Be gentle.**
❑ **Secure injured extremities.**

## *You can do it!*

# CHAPTER 11

## REEXAMINE

Your most important skill as a First Care Provider is your power of observation. Keep watching and rechecking Airway, Breathing, Circulation, and Spine. Also, after life support has been initiated and monitored, there is other important information that you may be able to gather.

## STAY WITH AND WATCH THE PATIENT

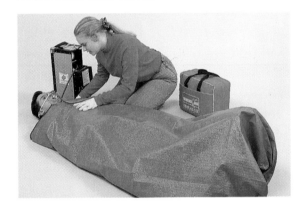

Stay with the patient and don't leave him alone except to call for help or vacate an area if you are in danger. Watch for indications of vomiting and be prepared to keep the airway open. Watch also for obvious changes in breathing and be sure to recheck any dressings or bandages.

## GET THE STORY

If time and circumstances permit, gather medical history information about the patient to pass along to the medical people. (You may be the last one to talk with a patient while he is still conscious.)

Ask a responsive person:

- What happened?
- What hurts/what's wrong?
- When did it start?
- Are you under a doctor's care?
- Do you take any medication? (Are you supposed to?)

Write down the answers to pass along to EMS or other appropriate people.

## LOOK FOR MEDICAL I.D.

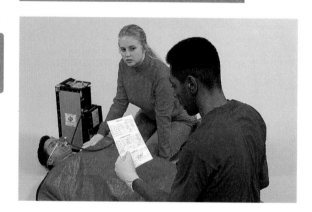

If the patient is unresponsive, determine if family, co-workers, or bystanders can provide any of this medical history. Also look for medical identification in the form of a medical warning bracelet, necklace, or a medical history form.

## MEASURE AND RECORD VITAL SIGNS

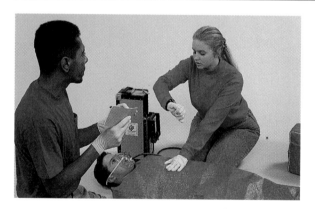

There are some important life function indicators that can help in measuring the effectiveness of your life support actions or the deterioration of the patient's condition. We call these indicators *vital signs*.

The three most important vital signs that can be readily measured are: *consciousness*, *heart rate*, and *breathing rate*.

If the situation permits or if you have someone to help in supporting the ABCS, measure and record a set of vital signs.

## Consciousness

Consciousness is one of the most basic functions of the brain. Loss of consciousness, even for a short period of time, can be a significant indicator of brain malfunction.

Measurement of consciousness is very simple:

- If someone responds to you, he is conscious.
- If there is no response, he is considered unconsciousness.

During First Care, why someone is unresponsive is not as important as the fact that they are.

## Breathing Rate

Most people take in and exhale air 12–20 times per minute. Depending on the nature and severity of a medical emergency, this rate can increase or decrease dramatically and result in serious consequences to the patient.

To measure someone's number of breaths per minute, simply watch the patient's chest and belly as it rises and falls. If necessary you can also place your hand on the upper belly/lower chest and feel the number of inhalations and exhalations.

## Pulse Rate

The human heart beats 70–90 times per minute. This rhythmic squeezing and relaxing creates blood pressure, which moves blood through the arteries to the brain and other body tissues.

There are many pulse points (in large arteries) where you can feel the pulsations created by the heart's beating. The most reliable is one of the two arteries in the neck.

Using two fingers (index and middle fingers), feel for the Adam's apple in the patient's neck; gently slide your finger into the groove next to the muscle alongside the neck. Press until you feel the heartbeat.

## SPECIAL POINT

When someone is conscious and aware that you are "counting breaths" they may become very self-conscious and alter their breathing rate. To adjust for this, have them close their eyes or, if possible, place an uninjured arm across their lower chest and "simulate" taking a wrist pulse as you are really feeling for breathing.

## CAUTION

Never feel both sides of the neck at the same time.

## Document Your Findings

If you determine vital signs, they will be of little value in establishing a baseline of the patient's condition and response to life support actions if you don't remember them and communicate them to medical responders. The emotions of the moment and your other important responsibilities could result in your forgetting the vital signs unless you write them down.

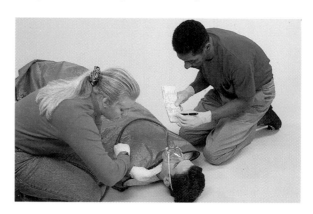

## VITAL SIGNS

| Date/Time | | | | | | | | | | | | |
|---|---|---|---|---|---|---|---|---|---|---|---|---|
| Conscious | Yes ☐ | No ☐ | Yes ☐ | No ☐ | Yes ☐ | No ☐ | Yes ☐ | No ☐ | Yes ☐ | No ☐ | Yes ☐ | No ☐ |
| Pulse Rate | | | | | | | | | | | | |
| Breathing Rate | | | | | | | | | | | | |

## REEXAMINE SUMMARY

❑ **Watch the patient's ABCS.**

❑ **Don't leave patient alone.**

❑ **Get the story of present and past medical problems.**

❑ **Measure and record vital signs.**

# *You can do it!*

# CHAPTER 12

## ENCOURAGE

You have a plan to follow to help control your emotions and emotional responses, but you will need to help the patient and bystanders deal with their emotions.

## EMOTIONAL SUPPORT

Most people confronted with what could be a life- or limb-threatening episode are going to have intense emotions—especially when it's his life and/or limb that is threatened.

Victims do not generally have a plan to follow, so their emotions may produce many intense emotional responses:

- Crying
- Yelling
- Nastiness
- Blank stare

All these reactions can significantly affect your attempt to help.

### Denial Is Not a River in Egypt

One of the most damaging emotional responses a seriously ill or injured person can experience is to deny the situation.

- "It's not happening."
- "There's nothing wrong with me."
- "I'm OK."

Denial is an ego defense mechanism that generally serves a good purpose. But in an emergency patient it can interfere with your attempt to help; a conscious patient states "I don't need any help," when it is quite obvious that he does. Don't be fooled by the patient.

Denial can be very annoying and cause you to abandon the patient. Recognition and persistence are the keys to dealing with denial and all other emotional responses.

## Don't Be "Taken In"

In dealing with an emergency patient's emotional responses, remember that as emotions increase, logic and sense of reality decrease. A patient's unpleasant or inappropriate emotional responses can easily trigger your own unacceptable response. Be careful not to overreact. The following behavior will help:

1. Speak softly but firmly. Yelling and screaming will only generate increased emotional response from your patient.

2. Don't threaten. The threat of physical harm or violence may well initiate a defensive act of violence on the part of an already out-of-control person. A slap on the face to help someone "get hold of himself" will most likely cause him to get hold of you.

3. Let the patient talk. An emotional patient needs to express her emotions, not suppress them. Don't stifle verbal communication. (Better out than in!) Your acceptance of her emotions gives her permission to start dealing with her feelings.

4. Be honest. Never lie to a patient. Don't tell them nothing's wrong when obviously there is a problem. But don't be brutally honest. They don't have to know how bad you think it is. Acknowledge that there is a problem and that you are doing all you can to help.

## Support the Will to Live

One of the most basic human instincts is the will to live. It is an innate drive to survive that kicks in at birth and continues throughout life. It's a known fact that people who lose the will to live usually die very soon thereafter.

Depending on the patient's perception of the severity of his problem and proximity to medical help, an emergency patient can give up hope.

Encourage and support the will to live by letting the patient know that you have First Care knowledge and skill, that you are going to help him until professional help arrives, and that he will do well.

## BYSTANDERS HAVE EMOTIONS TOO

Family members, co-workers, and even strangers who witness a medical emergency situation will also have intense emotions and exhibit emotional responses. These emotional responses can be very distracting as you attempt to provide initial life support. They can also be very alarming to the patient.

### Give Everyone Something to Do

Emotional intervention with bystanders is impossible while you are actively involved in life support actions. The best way to deal with emotional outbursts and irrational behavior is to channel the emotional energy of the bystanders. Give each a single positive action to keep them busy:

- "Go call 911."
- "Get me a blanket."
- "Hold the patient's chin up."
- "Keep the crowd back."

Remember, emotions are normal and very contagious. Avoid protracted discussions and arguments; they can quickly get out of hand in an emotionally charged atmosphere. Everyone at the scene of an emergency whose emotions go unchecked can significantly distract from your life support efforts.

## ENCOURAGE SUMMARY

❑ **Provide the patient emotional support.**
❑ **Support the patient's WILL TO LIVE.**
❑ **Watch what you say and how you say it.**
❑ **Channel bystander emotional energies by giving EVERYONE something to do.**

# *You can do it!*

# FIRST CARE CHEKSHEET™

## "QUIK CHEK"™

✓ **Check The Area**
☐ Hazards
☐ Latex Gloves
✓ **Do No Harm**
☐ Responsiveness?
✓ **Call Out for Help**
☐ Body Position
A – Airway
☐ Chin Position
☐ Obstruction
B – Breathing
☐ Look
☐ Listen
☐ Feel
✓ **Seek Medical Help ??**
C – Circulation
☐ Pulse
☐ Bleeding
S – Spine
☐ Mechanism of Injury
☐ Neck
☐ Head
☐ Limb Sensation
✓ **Support Life**
✓ **Make the Right Call (EMS) ???**

## ✓ Support Life

A ☐ Airway Maintained
☐ Mouth Cleared
☐ Heimlich Maneuver
☐ Positioned on Side ???
☐ Jaw Thrust
D ☐ Breathing Watched
☐ Oxygen _____ LPM
☐ Best Position _____
☐ Fresh Air
☐ Crowd Control
C ☐ Pulse Monitored
☐ Complete Rest
☐ Controlled Bleeding
☐ Where _____
☐ How _____
☐ Burns Cooled/Covered
☐ Legs Elevated
☐ Cover/Blanket
S ☐ Don't Move Patient/Parts
☐ Log Roll
☐ Immobilize Head

## *Until Help Arrives. . .*

C Communicate
☐ Talk to Patient
☐ Seek Medical Help
☐ Record Finding/Actions
☐ Advise/Supervisor/EMS

A Avoid Harm
☐ No Food/Drink
☐ Sugar (Diabetic?)
☐ No Medicine (MD?)
☐ Be Gentle
☐ Secure Body/Parts

R Re-examine
☐ Watch Patient (ABCS)
☐ Get the Story
☐ Info from Others?
☐ Medical I.D.?
☐ Measure Vital Signs?

E Encourage
☐ Emotional Support
☐ "Will to Live"
☐ Be Honest
☐ Watch What You Say
☐ Channel Energies

## *You can do it!*

# PART 4

## LIFE SUPPORT
## FOR SUDDEN DEATH

Cardiopulmonary resuscitation (CPR) was developed in the early 1960s in a major medical center in Baltimore, Maryland. It was created as a technique to help keep a patient's brain alive until sophisticated medical equipment could be brought to the bedside of someone whose heart suddenly stopped. It was learned that by "blowing" air into the patient's lungs and rhythmically "massaging" his chest, there was a dramatically better survival rate in sudden death patients waiting for the newly developed but very bulky defibrillator to be wheeled to the patient's room. This new technology could convert a life-threatening electrical malfunction in the heart into a normal rhythm.

In the thirty years since those days at John Hopkins University, dramatic advances in resuscitative medicine have continued: Defibrillators are now the size of a briefcase, and some models can be used by just about anyone; there are now drugs that, if administered soon enough, can dissolve the clots causing heart attacks and resulting in sudden death; open heart surgery can be performed to install new coronary artery pathways and in some instances even a new heart.

Yet all of these sophisticated and wonderful modern medical technologies are usually useless on someone whose heart stops and who does not immediately receive the simple life-supporting technique of CPR.

## YOU CAN HELP KEEP SOMEONE ALIVE

Remember, it takes time to die! When someone stops breathing and his heart stops beating, he is not really dead until his brain is dead. You can help keep such a person's brain alive by blowing air into his lungs and rhythmically pushing on his chest until advanced medical care is available. You can in fact provide the life-sustaining functions of Airway, Breathing, and Circulation by doing CPR.

# CHAPTER 13

## DOING CPR

## WHY CPR WORKS

The air we breathe contains about 21 percent of oxygen. With each breath we take this oxygen into our lungs, but normally we use only 5 percent of the oxygen inhaled; we exhale 16 percent back into the atmosphere. A person who isn't breathing can use the oxygen in our exhaled breath if we can gently force it into his lungs.

The heart beats because of the electrical signals from the brain. When these signals stop or when there are too many signals (fibrillation), the same end result occurs: No blood pressure is created to move oxygenated blood to the brain.

Because the heart is a flexible hollow organ, when stoppage or fibrillation occurs, you can rhythmically push and release on someone's chest to actually create enough blood pressure to send oxygenated blood to the brain and help keep it alive for several minutes. These chest compressions will squeeze the heart between the breastbone and the backbone. Such rhythmic squeezing, along with pressures in the chest, can create enough blood pressure to move blood to the lungs to pick up oxygen, return it back to the heart and then to the brain. Thus you can support life until professional medical care is available.

## HELPFUL BACKGROUND INFORMATION

The most common lethal complication involving the heart is an electrical malfunction known as fibrillation. Once in this erratic state, the heart receives and/or generates so many electrical impulses that it cannot effectively contract and relax to create the blood pressure necessary to circulate oxygenated blood.

A defibrillator is a device that sends an electrical current through the heart. This current can often shock the heart back into a normal, life-sustaining rhythm. Medical science has determined that fibrillation occurs in nearly all heart-attack-related-deaths.

With the advances of modern pre-hospital and hospital cardiac care and with the advent of fully automatic defibrillators, there is a greater opportunity to decrease the number of sudden deaths that deteriorate to brain death. Call EMS as soon as you determine that someone is in cardiac arrest. But don't stop there.

If a compact defibrillator (such as the one shown in the photo below) is readily available in your home or workplace, learn how to use it and apply it to anyone who is pulseless. However, even if such "rapid zap" technology is forthcoming, immediate CPR must be performed as soon as possible after someone collapses.

CPR and subsequent defibrillation don't always work. But as Dr. Safer has said, "They are the last, best hope for hearts and brains too good to die."

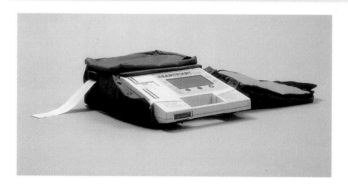

# THE EMERGENCY FIRST CARE PLAN FOR SUDDEN DEATH

When you find someone who has apparently collapsed, and your KSO says "UH-OH!"

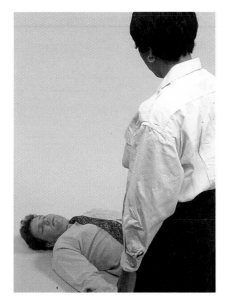

Check the area—be sure no harm will befall you.

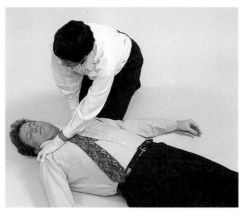

Attempt to rouse the person by gently shaking him and shouting something like, "Are you OK?"

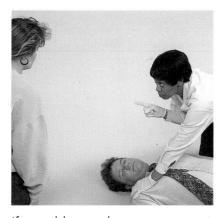

If possible, send someone to activate the EMS system or your medical response team.

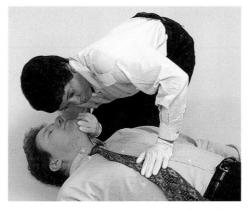

Determine the person's need for life support.

If your Quik Chek findings indicate the person is breathing and has a heartbeat, support Airway, Breathing, Circulation, and Spine. If you are alone and your Quik Chek indicates there is no Breathing, you must MAKE THE RIGHT CALL yourself. After calling, and until help arrives, you will have to provide ABCS.

# ADULT CPR

Doing CPR is as simple as ABC.

## A—Provide an Airway

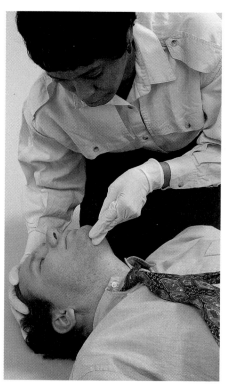

Gently push or pull up on the bony part of the patient' chin.

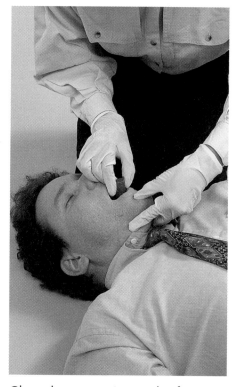

Clear the patient's mouth of anything you see that could later cause an airway problem (food, vomit, chewing gum, chewing tobacco, etc.).

## B—Provide Breaths

If you determine that the patient is not breathing, you will have to breathe for him (sometimes referred to as "artificial ventilation").

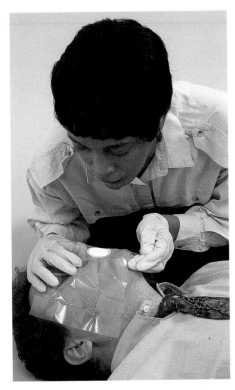

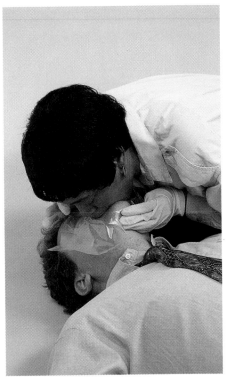

Pinch his nostrils to prevent air from escaping. While maintaining the chin lift, and placing mouth seal, place your mouth over his mouth. Be careful to make a tight seal.

Gently exhale into the patient's mouth until you see his chest rise.

Move your mouth away from the patient's mouth after the first breath and take a clean breath of air yourself; then give the patient a second breath as you did the first.

## C—Provide Circulation

If there is no pulse, be sure to place the patient on his back on a hard, flat surface (if he's not already there). This can be accomplished by carefully log-rolling a face-down person or, if the person is in a chair or on a bed, gently sliding him onto the floor. Be careful to protect his head and neck as best you can.

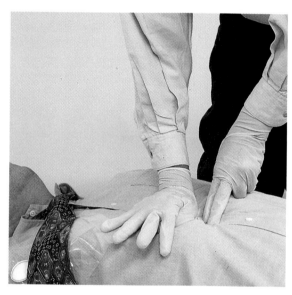

Kneel alongside him with your knees slightly apart for better balance. With two fingers of the hand closest to the person's waist, locate the rib cage. Feel along the edge of the last rib until you reach the notch at the bottom of the breastbone where both sides of the rib cage come together.

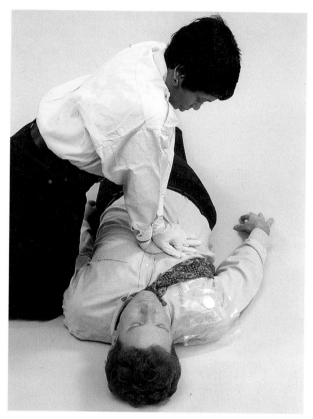

Place the heel of your other hand on the breastbone just above your two fingers. Now place your measuring hand on top of your other hand. Kneel up straight and lean over the patient, keeping your arms stiff and locking your elbows.

Compress the chest 1-1/2 to 2 inches deep. Repeat these compressions 15 times while maintaining a nice steady rhythm, allowing the same amount of time for compression as for relaxation.

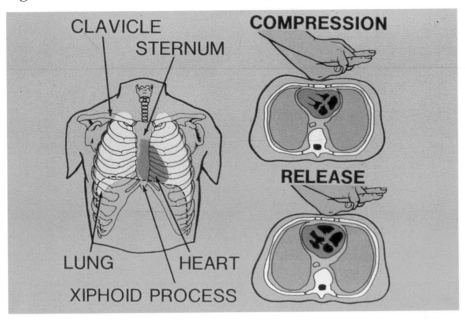

Give two more breaths as before (remember: not too hard or too fast) and then 15 more compressions. Repeat this cycle of 2 breaths/15 compressions.

Although it's highly unlikely that there will be a spontaneous return of the patient's own breathing and heart action, take five seconds to check for pulse and breathing after the first four or five cycles and every few minutes thereafter.

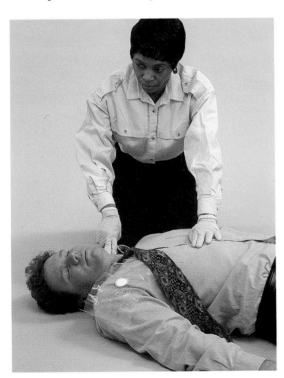

## Practice! Practice! Practice!

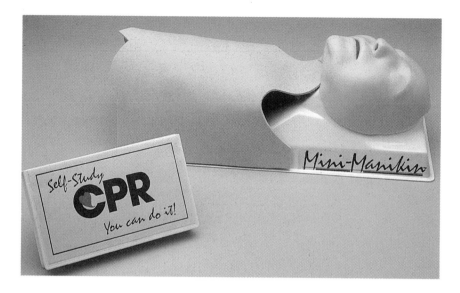

The best way to develop the confidence needed to actually perform CPR is to practice on a manikin. With new, inexpensive, and lightweight manikins such as Mini Manikin (shown above), you can even practice in the privacy of your own home.

You can also practice providing an airway and giving ventilations on a willing partner (and even practice hand and body positioning).

Remember as you do CPR:

1. Continue to CARE (Communicate, Avoid Harm, Reexamine, and Encourage).

2. Be sure help is on the way.

3. Be quick when checking for pulse and breathing return and try not to stop CPR for more than five seconds.

## IMPORTANT POINT

**Never** do actual chest compressions on anyone unless you are fairly certain that he does not have a pulse.

# CHAPTER 14

# CPR: ADDITIONAL FACTORS AND INFORMATION

The actual performance of life support procedures for the victim of cardiac arrest is quite simple. There are, however, some factors and circumstances that may affect your decision to act and the way in which you perform CPR.

## THE FACTS AND FIGURES

CPR doesn't always produce a desirable outcome. Depending on the state of health of the victim prior to collapse, the immediate cause of cardiac arrest, the time lapse between collapse and finding the person, how quickly you initiate life support actions, and the time it takes to administer advanced medical care, the patient may or may not survive. Based on these five variables, the survival rate of cardiac arrest victims varies widely (3–20 percent). If someone suffers a cardiac arrest and does not receive CPR within four minutes and advanced life support (drugs and defibrillation) within eight minutes, survival is extremely unlikely.

At the time of a cardiopulmonary arrest there is a very narrow window of opportunity for a desirable outcome. You, however, only control one and a half of the five variables. You can activate the EMS system (but you can't determine how quickly they will arrive) and you can provide effective CPR. It becomes absolutely essential, therefore, that you exercise what control you can or the patient has no chance for survival.

## MYTHS AND MISCONCEPTIONS

"CPR can save a life."

**JUST THE FACTS:**

CPR rarely, if ever, resuscitates or "brings someone back" from sudden death all by itself. It is a holding pattern to keep the brain alive until sophisticated paramedic or emergency department services can definitively intervene in the rapid progression from sudden death to brain death. But CPR can indeed keep someone alive and does play a vital part in the chain of survival. If you ever do CPR and the patient dies anyway, as sad and tragic as that will be, at least you can take comfort in the fact that you tried.

CPR doesn't always work, but at the time of a cardiac arrest you are faced with only two choices: (1) Possibly the person will live if you try CPR. (2) Definitely the person will die if you do nothing. Choose one!

## WHEN TO START CPR

The decision to start CPR is based on several basic indicators.

1. It is safe for you to be with and help the patient. Remember: You are not expected to die trying to give someone CPR.

2. The person looks terrible. Cardiac arrest victims are unresponsive and quickly lose normal skin color, appearing blue or gray. They may feel cold, often lose bowel and bladder control, and may have vomited.

3. As you perform a Quik Chek and look, listen, and feel for breathing, you find NO BREATHING.

4. When you check for a neck pulse for at least five to ten seconds you feel NO PULSE.

## WHEN TO STOP CPR

Continue doing CPR as best you can for as long as you can, and for as long as it is needed. Although the window of opportunity for success, as described previously, is very small, it is difficult to determine for certain that your efforts should end. In general, there are four situations that indicate you should stop CPR action.

1. *Patient's breathing and pulse return.* If, when you stop CPR to check for spontaneous breathing and a return of heartbeat, the patient appears to be breathing and circulating blood on her own, there is no need to continue CPR. (Clearly, if the patient wakes up and says "Thanks, I needed that," you shouldn't continue.)

   But in reality this rarely if ever occurs (except in the movies and on TV). The usual immediate cause of cardiac arrest—damage to heart muscle and/or electrical malfunction (fibrillation), cannot usually be helped or reversed by CPR alone. If, however, you are fortunate enough to witness the return of breathing and heartbeat, continue to check the ABCS continually: CARDIAC ARREST CAN OCCUR AGAIN.

2. *You are relieved by a qualified person.* If someone of equal or greater CPR ability and experience wants to take over, let her. Doing CPR is a physically and emotionally exhausting experience. Anyone else who can help, especially an EMS, medical, or public safety professional, is a welcome sight.

   There may even be situations when someone without any prior CPR knowledge or training can be taught on the spot to assist you in giving chest compressions, ventilations, or both. As long as such a person is willing and appears to be doing CPR as you are, let her help.

3. *Your own safety is in danger.* If, after you have initiated CPR, your own safety is compromised, remember the First Golden Rule: Self-survival! If there is a threat of violence, fire, turbulence, or any other situation in which you may be harmed, interrupt CPR. You are of no value to a patient in cardiac arrest if you become injured or dead.

4. *You are completely exhausted.* Again, CPR is a physically and emotionally demanding exercise. Initially your own adrenaline and body chemistry will kick in to give you the added strength needed to start CPR. But after a while, unless you are in great physical condition, you will tire and very probably begin to experience great pain in various parts of your body (e.g., back, arms, and knees).

   This is an added reason why you should call for help before you start CPR. But should it happen that you experience exhaustion before help arrives, stop CPR. You are not expected to be the next victim.

## Rescue Breathing

It is possible that a patient may not be breathing but does have a heartbeat. In this rare instance (possibly seen in the event of a drug overdose or near-drowning), there is no need to do full CPR. What you will have to do is simply provide one "artificial ventilation" every five seconds until help arrives or the patient breathes spontaneously. Between breaths, continue to monitor the patient's heart action by feeling for a pulse. (If the pulse stops, do full CPR.)

## WHEN NOT TO START CPR

There are several situations in which you need not do CPR on a pulseless, nonbreathing person (other than you being in immediate danger). Depending on local regulations, you need not start CPR if a terminally ill person has a "living will" in which she has requested no extraordinary life-prolonging measures or if a physician has issued a "No Code" or "Do Not Resuscitate" (DNR) order.

If a person is obviously dead beyond any hope of resuscitation, there is no reason to attempt CPR. Such situations include severing of the head from the body, decomposition of the body, or severe charring of the body from fire. The decision not to start CPR is always difficult and emotional. Death is never easy to deal with or accept, especially when it is the death of a loved one or close friend.

**If in doubt as to whether or not you should start CPR—start it!**

## KNOWING IF CPR IS EFFECTIVE

Short of the patient resuming spontaneous breathing and heart action (which, as indicated above, is very rare), it is difficult to determine exactly how effective are your CPR efforts. There are, however, some indicators to encourage you that your performance is supporting life.

If you see the chest rise or expand during ventilations you know that you're getting air into the lungs. Similarly, if a second rescuer can feel a neck pulse while you're delivering chest compressions to an otherwise pulseless person, there is a good likelihood that you are getting blood to the brain.

In some instances you may also detect a noticeable improvement in the patient's skin color; he may return closer to his normal skin tone. But if color does not return, this does not necessarily indicate ineffectiveness of getting "juice to the squash."

So by all means continue your actions as best you can for as long as you can.

## Ineffective CPR

There are a number of factors that could result in your CPR actions not being as effective as necessary to keep a person in cardiac arrest "brain alive" until help arrives. It is important that you give the best CPR you can under the circumstances. Consideration of these factors could have a significant effect on the outcome of your life support efforts.

1. Patient not on a firm surface.

   If the patient is on a bed, couch, or other such soft surface it will be difficult to effectively compress the chest between the breastbone and backbone and create the necessary pressure to move blood to the brain.

2. Poor mouth seal.

   There must be a firm seal between your lips and the patient's mouth, or your exhaled air will leak out around the patient's face and not go into his lungs.

3. Poor or no chin lift.

   Failure to open the airway will result in less-than-adequate ventilations. Remember that the tongue is attached to the jaw. In a sudden death patient the jaw relaxes, causing the tongue to slide back or partially block the airway. If the chin is not properly lifted, the tongue may prevent air from going into the lungs.

4. Improper hand position.

   For the chest to be most effectively compressed, your hands must be midline and on the lower half of the breastbone. The force of your compressions ideally should be delivered to this single spot. Pressure anywhere else on the chest wall could result in possible internal injury and, more importantly, inadequate circulation.

5. Improper strokes.

   Compressing the chest too hard or too fast will not allow the heart the proper time to empty and refill again. It will also tire you too quickly. The downstroke of each compression should take as long as the upstroke; both should be in a nice, steady rhythm. Counting out loud helps to maintain this smooth action.

## COMPLICATIONS OF CPR

Even if done optimally, CPR can and often does produce complications. In your efforts to support life, you may inadvertently cause broken ribs, a bruised heart, and soft tissue injury around the patient's mouth. Doing CPR as described here will greatly reduce these complications but probably not eliminate them. Nevertheless, survivors of cardiac arrest have gladly complained of these complications.

One of the most common complications is that the patient will vomit. Air entering the stomach combined with chest compressions can result in emptying of the stomach contents.

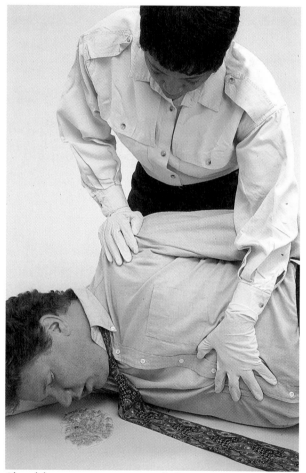

Should vomiting occur, roll the patient onto either side and clear his mouth as best you can. Then reposition the patient on his back and continue CPR.

CPR is not an exact science, and it is most often provided under intense emotional stress. (Over 90 percent of the time a First Care Giver administers CPR it is to a family member, a loved one, or a close friend.) Remember, the worst complication of all is a death that occurs because no one attempted the life support actions of CPR. Perfect CPR is virtually nonexistent. Good CPR is desirable and acceptable. But *ANY CPR IS BETTER THAN NO CPR.*

## Catching Things

Of all emergency medical procedures, doing CPR involves the most intimate and personal contact with another human being. This direct contact with the body (and very often body fluids) of another person brings with it understandable concern about the communication of disease from the victim to the rescuer.

The possibility of a CPR provider catching any disease from the patient is extremely low. There are no reported incidences of AIDS or any other fatal diseases being transmitted during CPR. Although the threats may be limited, the fears are very real. Attention must be paid to insuring your personal health and safety when administering CPR to anyone.

## HELPFUL BACKGROUND INFORMATION

Infectious diseases are illnesses that are communicated by microscopic organisms generally classified as either bacteria or viruses. These organisms usually enter the body via a variety of routes of transmission: breaks in the skin, respiratory tract, the digestive system, direct blood contact, or mucus membrane linings (such as those inside sex organs).

Once in the body, these microbes can dramatically reproduce and multiply, attacking tissue of various body organs and/or interfering with the function of infected body systems.

Not everyone who has disease-causing viruses or bacteria enter their body will develop a disease. Whether or not disease-causing microbes will affect a previously uninfected individual will depend on a variety of factors, including age, preexisting illness, the quantity of organisms transmitted, frequency of exposure, and ultimately, the ability of an individual's immune system to destroy and/or neutralize invading organisms.

Because disease-developing variables are difficult to quantify or verify prior to exposure, it makes good sense to eliminate contact with these organisms and to limit or shield the most common routes of entry.

Wearing latex gloves, using a barrier between your mouth and that of the sudden death patient, and proper hand washing afterward are the best-known ways of universal precaution during and after giving CPR.

## USE OF CPR BREATHING DEVICES

Devices used to deliver ventilations during CPR fall into two main categories: face shields and face masks. Both have advantages and disadvantages and are most effective when the user has prior knowledge and training in the use of specific devices.

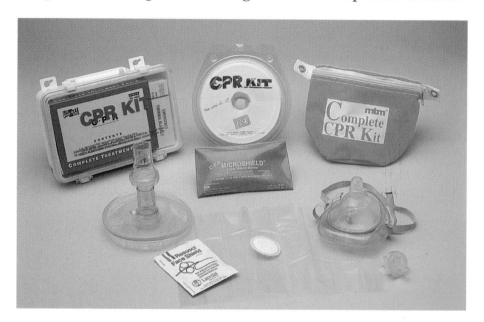

To use a mask-type device the rescuer must make a tight seal between the face of the patient and the device. *Caution*: Because such action will tend to close the airway, the First Care Giver must also simultaneously lift up on the patient's chin to keep the victim's tongue away from the back of his throat.

Many CPR devices are equipped with a one-way valve mechanism to prevent the patient's exhaled air or secretions from entering the CPR provider's mouth. Some devices also allow for the attachment of an oxygen unit to provide greater oxygen content to each ventilation during CPR.

Generally, when using a mask, the device will cover the patient's nose and mouth and the patient's nose need not be squeezed. Once the device is in place and the airway maintained, simply blow into the top of the device. A shield-type device will usually require that you pinch the nose before giving breaths. As with mouth-to-mouth ventilation, providing breaths to a patient through a device should not be done too hard and only until the chest rises.

Commercially available face-shield devices are generally a plastic material with an opening or membrane that permits air to go from your mouth to the nonbreathing patient's. You can also improvise such a device with a cloth, handkerchief, or napkin. The patient's nose must still be squeezed and the air exchange point must be over the patient's mouth. Using a breathing bag device (such as that shown in illustration below) is not recommended for First Care Givers. Such devices require intensive training and frequent utilization to maintain proficiency. Furthermore, unless the patient has a tube placed directly into his lungs via the windpipe (a skill well beyond the ability of a First Care Giver), it has been shown that this device frequently does not deliver enough air into the lungs.

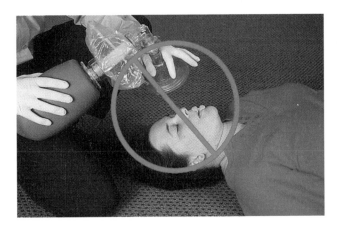

Another device to definitely avoid is an oxygen-powered resuscitator. These very heavy and very expensive units are also very dangerous and virtually useless in the hands of First Care Providers.

# CHAPTER 15

## SPECIAL CPR PATIENTS AND SITUATIONS

There are a few circumstances where providing life support for apparent sudden death will require creative or modified application of CPR and/or some additional actions.

### DOING CPR IN DIFFICULT LOCATIONS

You are not expected to start CPR if there is a significant danger present (e.g., fire, highway traffic, or waves over the bow of a ship), nor should you continue CPR if your own safety is threatened after you initiate life support action.

There are other situations in which you decide to initiate CPR, but the physical circumstances may necessitate that you be somewhat creative or innovative. In short, you may have to vary CPR performance slightly to accomplish the goal of helping keep the brain alive.

In a confined space, for example, you may not be able to position yourself directly over the person's chest to do chest compressions. Another example is in a commercial airplane where you may well need to stop CPR and buckle-up during the deceleration of landing.

Also, depending on space, it may take two people to do one-person CPR. In the past two-person CPR was routinely taught; however, data has shown it rarely worked and often caused too much confusion for nonmedical personnel. Nevertheless, in certain locations—for example, in the aisle of a commercial airplane—it could be virtually impossible for one person alone to pump the chest and then reposition to ventilate the lungs. In such instances, two people may need to do "One Person CPR," maintaining the 15-to-2 ratio of chest compressions to ventilations.

In summary, if you can safely initiate CPR, do it as best you can under the circumstances in which you find yourself.

# CHILD AND INFANT CPR

Children are not miniature adults. Although the rationale and principles of CPR for children are the same as for adults, their size and some body structure differences necessitate a few modifications in applying CPR techniques.

Children generally have healthy and strong hearts, undamaged by smoking and dietary abuse. If cardiac arrest occurs in kids, it is usually due to accidents such as drowning or suffocation, or more likely as a result of progressive breathing difficulty. It is therefore very important to identify infants and children with breathing compromise and to intervene with breathing support as soon as possible. Should they need CPR or "resusci-breathing," the following special actions and considerations should be followed.

## Infant CPR (Birth to one year of age)

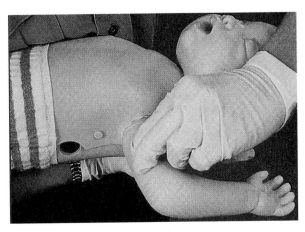

Feel for pulse on inside of upper arm.

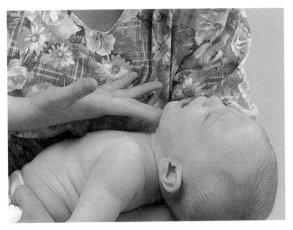

Do not overextend the infant's head or neck. Place your mouth over the infant's nose and mouth and give only a "puff" of breath.

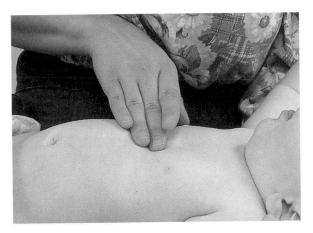

Use two fingers to do chest compressions over center of breastbone. Compress five times, 1/2–1 inch deep, one finger width below an imaginary "nipple line."

The CPR rate for infants is five compressions and then one breath until help arrives.

## Child CPR (One to eight years of age)

Place your mouth over child's mouth (or mouth and nose if possible) and gently ventilate until you see the chest rise (*NOT fill*). Use only one hand to do chest compressions (1–1-1/2 inches deep).

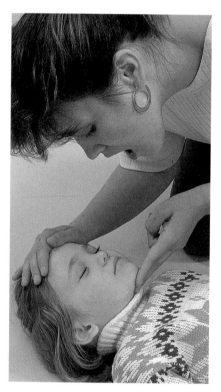 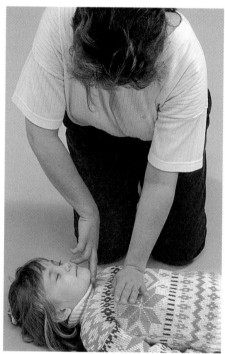

The CPR rate for children is five compressions and then one breath until help arrives.

## NEAR DROWNING

In the case of a near-drowning situation, your Emergency First Care plan remains the same. Safely remove the victim from the water. (Remember: If you can't swim, don't jump into the water yourself.) Then perform a Quik Chek, Make The Right Call (or send someone else to call EMS), and then perform CPR or rescue breathing, depending on which is needed.

Don't worry about the small amount of water that may be in the lungs. Death from drowning is caused by asphyxiation (no air in the lungs), not from water in the lungs. In fact, drowning and near-drowning victims usually have very little water in their lungs.

Near-drowning victims have a better-than-average chance of being revived by CPR because cold water lowers the brain's need for oxygen, and because generally they begin with healthy hearts. Should a near-drowning victim begin breathing on his own, it is very important that he be placed under medical care. It is not uncommon for near-drowning survivors to develop serious lung complications within 24–48 hours.

## COLD ENVIRONMENT

If an apparently dead, stiff body is discovered in a very cold environment, the victim may be suffering from hypothermia. In such a patient, core body temperature is extremely low and the heartbeat and breathing may be absent or impossible to determine.

In hypothermia the brain's need for oxygen is greatly diminished and it takes longer for brain death to occur. Therefore, don't presume that a patient is beyond help. Begin CPR and continue your resuscitation efforts until medical rewarming can be accomplished. There is nothing a First Care Giver can or should do to rewarm a cardiac arrest victim outside of a medical facility.

## NECK BREATHERS

Someone who has had his voice box surgically removed no longer breathes through his mouth and nose; he breathes through a hole in the throat called a stoma.

Performing mouth-to-mouth ventilations on someone who has had this procedure (known as a laryngectomy) will be useless. In order to breathe air into the lungs of such a patient, you must do mouth-to-stoma ventilations when doing CPR or rescue breathing.

**IMPORTANT POINT**

A hypothermic victim is not dead until he is warm and dead.

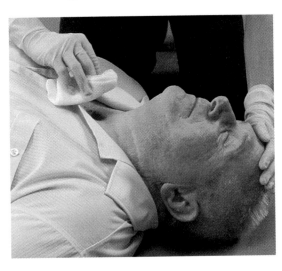

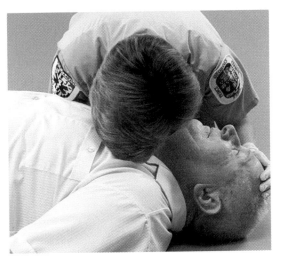

# OBSTRUCTED AIRWAY (UNRESPONSIVE PATIENT)

If someone who is choking collapses, or if you are unable to get any air into an unconscious nonbreathing patient, he may well have an airway obstructed by food or some other object. In either case, you won't know whether the airway is blocked until you attempt to ventilate. if you do not see the chest rise during ventilations, you will have to use a modified Heimlich maneuver on the patient to help remove the possible obstruction.

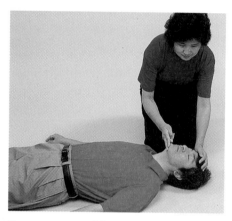

If you are unable to ventilate a non-breathing patient successfully, attempt to reposition the airway and again try to breathe for the patient again.

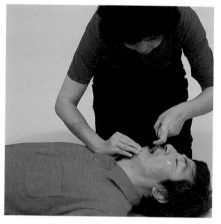

Perform a finger sweep throughout the patient's mouth to see if you dislodged the obstruction.

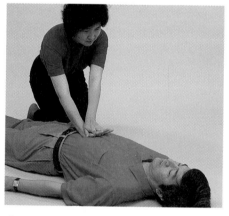

If you are still unsuccessful, reposition your body and push in five times at the same spot where you would have squeezed up and in to perform the Heimlich maneuver. (Kneel alongside the patient or straddle her.)

Repeat the sequence of two attempts at ventilation, five abdominal thrusts, a one-finger sweep ("Rule 251") until the object is dislodged or you can ventilate the patient.

# DON'T LET IT HAPPEN TO YOU!

Although many factors can cause sudden heart stoppage, by far the most common cause of sudden death is complications due to heart problems. Sadly, these precipitating heart problems rarely are "sudden." Many of the victims of heart attacks (and even some who have survived cardiac arrest) confess to days, and sometimes weeks, of ignored symptoms.

## Warning Signs of a Serious Heart Problem

- Chest pain, pressure, or discomfort usually lasting more than two minutes
- Pain in arms, neck, jaw, or back
- Lightheadedness or weakness
- Nausea and/or sweating
- Denial that anything is wrong

In general, listen to your body. If on more than one occasion pain or discomfort develops during specific activities but then eases or disappears in a short period of time, tell your doctor. Be especially alert to a pattern of unusual chest sensations which occur:

- At rest or during sleep
- At varying levels of exertion
- At specific times of the day (especially upon awakening)
- Upon exposure to cold temperatures
- Under emotional stress

Be aware of these warning signs and don't allow denial to overpower reason. Get medical help. Better to be wrong about your suspicion than "dead right."

# FIRST CARE CHEKSHEET™

## Life Support *for "Sudden Death"*

√ **Check The Area/Latex Gloves???**

☐ Establish Unresponsiveness

☐ Yell Out for Help

☐ Body Position ???

☐ Open Airway

☐ Look, Listen, Feel for Breathing

☐ Make the Right Call (EMS) ???

☐ Place Face Shield/Mask ???

☐ Pinch Nostrils ???

☐ Give 2 Slow Breaths (not too hard)

☐ Feel for a Pulse

☐ Patient on Firm Surface

☐ Locate Hand Position

☐ Position Your Body/Lock Your Elbows

☐ Give 15 Chest Compressions ($1\frac{1}{2}$–2 in. deep)

☐ Repeat 2 Breaths (see chest rise)

☐ Continue Compressions and Ventilations . . .

**Continue CPR care until:**

1. Patient's breathing and pulse return.

2. You are relieved by a qualified person.

3. Your own safety is in danger.

4. You are completely exhausted.

## *You can do it!*

# PART 5

## PUTTING IT ALL TOGETHER

Whether you respond to a medical emergency at home, work, or elsewhere in your community, your decision to provide Emergency First Care requires knowledge, skills, and control of emotional response. But your life support actions will also require a well-defined support structure including various human and material resources as well as evaluation of your performance. That planned structure is your Emergency Medical Response System.

# CHAPTER 16

## DEVELOPING AN EMERGENCY MEDICAL RESPONSE SYSTEM

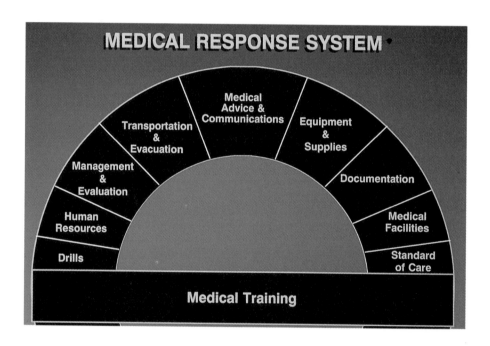

MEDICAL RESPONSE SYSTEM

Medical Advice & Communications

Transportation & Evacuation

Equipment & Supplies

Management & Evaluation

Documentation

Human Resources

Medical Facilities

Drills

Standard of Care

Medical Training

## STANDARD OF CARE

The Standard of Care is the sum total of actions you are expected to take at the time of a potential medical emergency. As an average person who has not chosen the provision of medical services as your life's work (and even if you are a member of a health profession), if you are the first to detect and respond to someone with a sudden medical problem, you are not expected to "heal nor cure" that person.

What is expected of you, and what you should expect of yourself, is that you generally follow the Emergency First Care plan and ABCS CARE actions, as outlined in this book, as best you can under the circumstances. In essence, your standard of care is to Support Life: ABCS—Check 'em and make 'em the best they can be.

## CASE EVALUATION

Did you do a good job? At the time of a medical emergency and afterward, it's only natural that you will want to evaluate your performance. After all, everyone wants to do good and no one wants to make mistakes, especially if those mistakes can result in greater harm to another person.

But bear in mind that your evaluation of yourself should be based only on process—did you follow the ABCS CARE steps as best you could under the circumstances?—not on outcome or results.

---

### MYTHS AND MISCONCEPTIONS

"You determine if someone lives or dies at the time of a medical emergency."

**JUST THE FACTS:**

"The operation was a success but the patient died" is an old and not-very-funny joke. But it makes an important point. The outcome of a medical procedure is not determined by the actions of a doctor, hospital, or First Care Giver alone.

Outcome following a medical emergency is determined by four vital factors:

1. The victim or patient's state of health prior to the event.
2. The seriousness of the event or mechanism of injury.
3. The timely response and quality of the EMS and medical-care systems.
4. The life support actions of the first person to detect and attend to the perceived medical problem.

Because you can only control the last of these crucial variables, whether or not an outcome is desirable or undesirable is not within your control. It is only the process of life support for which you can be held accountable.

---

## You Can Make the Difference

Your actions can make a positive difference in the outcome, but they may not. If someone needs life support assistance and you do nothing, what chances for survival he had are greatly diminished. If you give the best care you can under the circumstances, his chances are significantly improved.

If you give someone proper Emergency First Care and he survives, you can enjoy credit for that result (and remind him of that fact every time you see him!). If despite your best efforts someone dies, it will hurt a great deal, even if you didn't know that person prior to the emergency event. But at least you will have the comfort of knowing you did everything possible to help.

## LEGAL CONSIDERATIONS

Being sued is a major fear for some people when they face an event requiring them to give Emergency First Care. Despite many rumors and horror stories to the contrary, the legal system protects the person who volunteers to help at the time of a medical emergency. The fear of litigation is generally much greater than the actual threat.

However, since according to our legal system it could theoretically happen, we need to examine several issues.

### Duty to Give Emergency Care

Traditionally, common law does not mandate that a person must provide emergency care to another person in need of it unless there is an explicit statute, regulation, or contractual obligation to do so. Doctors, nurses, and paramedics performing their normal work responsibilities have a duty to patients for whom they are caring.

Many nonmedical-service employers have a regulatory requirement to make initial emergency care available in their workplaces. Acting as an agent of your employer, you may have a responsibility to render appropriate reasonable care in your workplace until medical help arrives.

In some states, drivers are required by law to stop at roadside accidents and render aid. Other states require citizens to stop and render assistance to any person exposed to grave physical harm (especially in highway accident situations).

Whatever your motivation or obligation, if you offer to help it could well be construed that you have incurred a duty to provide reasonable care at that time.

## Consent

If the victim of a potential medical emergency is conscious, you should inform her of your intentions and seek her approval before touching her or giving any aid. A simple "I've had Emergency First Care training, can I help you?" will suffice. The person does, however, have the right to refuse help.

As frustrating as a refusal of help may be for you (especially when it's obviously a serious problem), all you can do is be persistent in your willingness to help. Be careful not to become aggressive or antagonistic, as this may further delay care.

If someone is unconscious or otherwise unresponsive, it is obviously not possible to obtain voiced consent. In such instances you can assume "implied consent" and may proceed to offer initial care. The courts presume that the average intelligent person wants to live and would, if they could, willingly accept reasonable help.

## Be Reasonable

Regardless of your motivation or obligation to give care to someone in need, society and the courts expect that you will do so according to the principle of the *reasonably prudent person.* Simply stated, this legal standard means that you will conduct yourself as any ordinary person (with similar knowledge, skills, and training) would act in a comparable emergency situation.

Any individual who gives emergency care need only exercise reasonable care under the circumstances. To act in an unreasonable manner could be construed as a breach of duty (or negligence) and subject you to legal liability. What is reasonable is measured by your level of training and experience as well as the circumstances surrounding the emergency.

Many people express the belief that often in life "you are damned if you do and damned if you don't." The greatest potential for a lawsuit against a company or employer occurs when nothing is done to help a patient despite the fact that reasonable care is available. Therefore, do something—but do the right thing. Your best defense against legal action (for you or your company) is ABCS CARE!

With regard to any other emergency medical action or procedure not described in this book, unless you are specifically trained, equipped, and authorized to provide such care, don't do it!

## Damages and Cause

For you to be sued or held liable in an emergency case where you had a duty to give reasonable care, the patient must have sustained actual measurable damages. Furthermore, such damage must be a direct result (proximate cause) of your negligent actions.

In the case of providing CPR to a person who suffers sudden death, it is virtually impossible to do harm to an already dead person. If a still-living patient or a CPR survivor sustains an injury as a result of your care (e.g., a broken rib) it would have to be shown that your care procedures were not reasonable.

When providing Emergency First Care, to limit liability and legal action, provide ABCS CARE or CPR (when needed) as best you can under the circumstances.

## Good Samaritan Laws

Virtually all states have enacted legislation known as Good Samaritan laws to protect certain persons from civil damages as a result of harm caused to an emergency patient by their actions or ordinary negligence. Many such statutes cover only physicians and nurses; in some states the statute has been extended to policeman, firemen, and paramedical personnel. A few states extend such protection to all citizens.

The intent of Good Samaritan legislation was to encourage those who could give lifesaving care to do so for someone in need without fear of civil liability. However, Good Samaritan laws do not cover anyone with a duty to provide care who expects to be compensated for his service.

## HUMAN RESOURCES

People are the reason for establishing a Medical Response System; people operate and manage it. All persons employed at a particular work site potentially play a part in the established Medical Response System.

Management responsibilities, levels of training, and personal experience will determine individual emergency response and life support roles and functions. Generally, those employees trained as Emergency First Care Providers will have key roles in their company's Medical Response System.

Establishing an Emergency Response Team is a proven method to effectively prepare and manage available human resources and to deliver appropriate emergency care at a work site. Based on the total number of workers, particular dangers or hazards, and the likelihood and frequency of serious incidents occurring, the structure and function of an Emergency Response Team may vary.

In some workplaces the Emergency Response Team has responsibilities for fire, rescue, and other emergency situations as well as for serious medical events. In others, there may be a separate Medical Response Team based on individual interests and temperament. Regardless of the structure, there are many benefits to having such teams.

In addition to delivering a consistent standard of care for ill or injured co-workers, an Emergency Response Team can significantly improve overall company team spirit and morale. The creation of such teams also demonstrates management commitment to a safe and healthful work environment.

However, it must be noted that except at the time of an actual medical emergency, establishment and operation of such teams must not be allowed to interfere with the daily course of business of a company. The primary responsibility of Emergency Response Team members is to produce the product or deliver the service for which they were hired and for which their company or agency receives payment or funding. Preparing for and/ or providing emergency care when needed is but a humanitarian gesture and an adjunct responsibility.

## EMERGENCY CARE TRAINING

Specific medical response and life support training programs should be provided to all appropriate individuals. The content and duration of such training depend on the established standard of care and the likelihood of maintaining proficiency of needed life support skills.

There are numerous training programs and materials available for instructing medical and nonmedical personnel in basic emergency care skills. Determining which is best for your particular needs will require some planning and analysis. To assist you in evaluating a particular program, we offer the "Seven C's" checklist.

### Capabilities

- What is the standard of care expected at your location or work site?
- Does the curriculum have reasonable and appropriate behavioral objectives? (i.e., a plan of action)
  1. Recognize that there may be a problem.

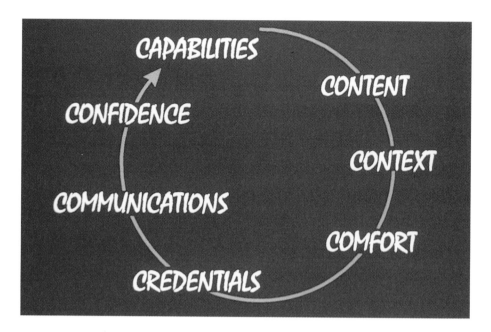

2. Decide to take action.

3. Assess the status of Airway, Breathing, and Circulation, and possibility of Spine injury.

4. Know how and when to summon appropriate help.

5. Provide life support until help arrives.

## Content

- Is the content based on the capabilities and specific care skills to be developed?
- Does the curriculum contain unnecessary or complicated medical detail?
- Does the curriculum present information on recognizing and dealing with emotions at the time of an emergency event?

## Context

- Does the curriculum address the particular needs and temperament of the targeted audience?
- Does the curriculum consider the location and environment in which students are likely to use their life support skills?
- Does the curriculum consider the likelihood of skills degradation?

## Communication

- Do programs follow proven educational principles? (i.e., Tell, Show, Do, Review)

- Is instructor emphasis on learning, not teaching?
- Is appropriate use made of audiovisuals and hands-on sessions?

## Comfort

- Is training provided in a physically comfortable and nonintimidating setting?
- Is there ample space for hands-on practical skills sessions?
- Do audiovisuals avoid use of graphic "gore and guts" illustrations and intimidating medical terminology?
- Do program materials and presentations contain appropriate use of humor?

## Credentials

- Have appropriate governmental and medical authorities recognized the training program?
- Are programs conducted by experienced individuals who have completed special instructor training?
- If instructors are nonmedical professionals, have they been trained by clinically experienced and educationally qualified EMS or health care professionals?
- Are program attendees given written recognition for their participation in the program?

## Confidence

- Are program goals achievable?
- Do participants develop a sense of accomplishment?
- Can acquired skills be maintained?

## COMMUNICATIONS TECHNOLOGY

Communications technology is an integral part of your Medical Response System. Normally it is through telephone, radio, or satellite communications that you will access EMS or other medical service support and assistance.

It is important, therefore, that you keep your communications equipment in good working condition (including freshly charged batteries, if needed) and that you are familiar with how to use it.

It is also vital that you plan in advance where you are going to call by posting emergency phone numbers (or radio frequencies and call letters) on or near your communications equipment.

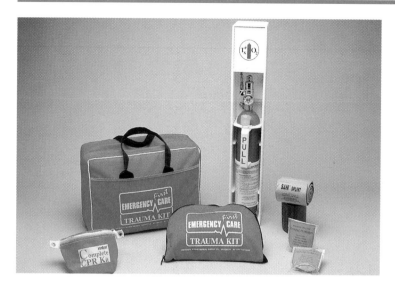

In general, you need very little or no specialized equipment to give Emergency First Care. Your most important emergency care "devices" are your hands, your mouth, and your brain.

Nevertheless, a few items can be assembled and kept in your Emergency First Care kit. These include:

ROLLER BANDAGES
ACE BANDAGE
TRIANGULAR BANDAGES
ADHESIVE TAPE
STERILE GAUZE DRESSINGS (4" X 4")
PROTECTIVE BLANKETS
COLD PACK (CHEMICAL)
STERILE WATER (FOR IRRIGATION)
PEN LIGHT
TRAUMA SCISSORS
LATEX GLOVES
CPR MASK OR FACE SHIELD
HAND-CLEANSING TOWELETTES
PEN OR PENCIL
FIRST CARE CHECKLIST

The items suggested are minimum only. Additional items may be included to suit your individual needs.

Rather than create your own kit, you may choose to purchase a commercially available one. But use caution in selecting an off-the-shelf unit: Many first aid kits contain inappropriate items and supplies (bite stick, ointments, tourniquets, "eye magnets," etc.), while others contain useless filler and unnecessary materials which drive up the price.

## DOCUMENTATION

Keeping a written record of your findings and actions in an emergency medical situation is a vital component of your Medical Response System. Proper documentation serves three essential purposes.

**Emergency Care Actions.**   Writing down your findings and actions is one of the best ways for you to remember to complete all of the necessary ABCS CARE steps. A checklist such as the one shown will remind you to perform all potentially needed life support procedures and will provide a written record for future reference.

**Continuing the Process of Care.**   Such a written document should also be given to EMS or other medical personnel who take over from you. This will provide medical personnel with a detailed description of the patient's condition from as early on in the event as possible. It will also convey to them what care you provided and the patient's response, if any, to those actions.

**Legal Protection.**   Although the likelihood of litigation against a First Care Giver is extremely remote, a written description of your findings and actions is an important part of your defense should legal action against you or your employer arise following an emergency medical situation.

Regardless of your intentions, actions, or memory, in medical and legal circles it is a well-established dictum, "If it wasn't written down it wasn't done."

# FIRST CARE CHEKSHEET™

✓ **Check The Area**
☐ Hazards
☐ Latex Gloves
✓ **Do No Harm**
☐ Responsiveness?
☐ Body Position
**A** – Airway
☐ Chin Position
☐ Signs of Obstruction
**B** – Breathing
☐ Look
☐ Listen
☐ Feel
✓ **Call for Help ???**
**C** – Circulation
☐ Pulse
☐ Bleeding
**S** – Spine
☐ Mechanism of Injury
☐ Neck
☐ Head
☐ Limb Sensation

✓ **Support Life**
**A** ☐ Airway Maintained
　☐ Mouth Cleared
　☐ Heimlich Maneuver
　☐ Positioned on Side ???
　☐ Jaw Thrust ???
**B** ☐ Breathing Watched
　☐ Oxygen
　☐ Best Position _____
　☐ Fresh Air
　☐ Crowd Control
**C** ☐ Pulse Checked
　☐ Complete Rest
　☐ Controlled Bleeding
　☐ Where _____
　☐ How _____
　☐ Burns Cooled/Covered
　☐ Legs Elevated ???
　☐ Cover/Blanket
**S** ☐ Don't Move Patient
　☐ Immobilize Head
　☐ Log Roll ???
　☐ Collar/Spine Board ???

✓ **CPR**
*(for "Sudden Death")*
If no breathing/pulse. . .
☐ Phone for Help ???
☐ Body Position ???
☐ Open Airway
☐ Place Face Shield/
　Mask ???
☐ Pinch Nostrils ???
☐ Give 2 Slow Breaths
　(not too hard)
☐ Patient on Firm Surface
☐ Locate Hand Position
☐ Position Your Body
☐ Give 15 Chest
　Compressions
　(1½–2 in. deep)
☐ Repeat Cycle
　(15 Compressions:
　2 Breaths)

✓ *Until Help Arrives. . .*
**C** – Communicate
　☐ Talk to Patient
　☐ Make the Right Call
　☐ Record Care
　☐ Advise Team/Supervisor
**A** – Avoid Harm
　☐ No Food/Drink
　☐ Sugar (Diabetic?)
　☐ No Medicine (MD?)
　☐ Be Gentle
　☐ Secure Body/Parts
**R** – Re-Examine
　☐ Watch Patient (ABCS)
　☐ Get the Story (over)
　☐ Don't Leave Alone
　☐ Measure Vital Signs (over)
**E** – Encourage
　☐ Emotional Support
　☐ "Will to Live"
　☐ Be Honest
　☐ Watch What You Say
　☐ Channel Energies

*You can do it!*

© 1996 Emergency & Safety Programs, Inc., 00 Main Street, Chester, PA 19015 • (610) 872-7447

# PROFESSIONAL MEDICAL SERVICES

It is the objective of Emergency First Care to control complications and provide life support to seriously ill or injured persons until professional medical care is available, that is, until the next level of the EMS system can take over.

Usually it will not be your decision which level or which service to "hand off to." At work you may have a staffed medical department on site. In the community the EMS dispatcher will often select which type of prehospital care unit (Basic EMT or Advanced Paramedic) will respond. If the situation is apparently serious or life-threatening, the ambulance personnel will usually decide to which hospital or specialty center (e.g. trauma, burn, cardiac, etc.) the patient will be transported.

But there may be times when the First Care Giver may have to make the choice as to which type or level of services is needed. It is important, therefore, for you to be familiar with the emergency medical resources available to you in your community.

## IMPORTANT BACKGROUND INFORMATION

### Who's Who in EMS?

There are many individuals on the community EMS team. In some areas titles, qualifications, and training vary slightly, but here are some general descriptions of key personnel:

**Dispatcher.**   Dispatchers are specially trained to determine the type of emergency the caller is reporting and to alert appropriate medical and public safety responders. Often, they direct the person in providing care until help arrives. The dispatcher must also keep track of available units, inform them of the nature and location of a call, and communicate to them any information regarding patient status or condition.

**First Responder.**   First Responders are generally the first public safety professionals to arrive at an emergency call. They could be the police, a rescue unit, or the fire department. Their training consists of at least 40 hours of basic life support skills, emergency vehicle response, emergency scene procedures, and assisting medical units.

**EMT.**   EMTs (Emergency Medical Technicians) are trained in noninvasive life support and ambulance operations. Often they are teamed with paramedics. Along with 100-plus hours of basic life support training, EMTs are trained in vehicle extrication and how to assist paramedics in advanced medical care.

**Paramedic.**   Paramedics are highly trained in providing the advanced medical care (starting IVs, reading EKGs, defibrillating, etc.) needed to support the life of critically ill or injured persons. Initially trained as EMTs, paramedics attend 6 to 24 months of additional professional training.

**Flight Nurse.**   Flight nurses are often the "team leaders" on medical helicopter flight crews. Often they are emergency or critical care nurses with two to four years of education plus special training in in-flight physiology and the care of critically injured persons at the scene.

**Certified Emergency Nurse.**   Registered nurses with advanced training in emergency care, Certified Emergency Nurses have passed a rigorous national exam. CENs have many responsibilities in the emergency department. They evaluate each person's condition to determine who should be seen first, must coordinate the care of patients with many types of illnesses and injuries, assist the Emergency Physician and/or medical specialist, and deal with family members.

**Emergency Physician.**   Generally having completed a three-year residency after medical school, Emergency Physicians are specialists in all aspects of medicine, with special emphasis on emergency medicine.

**Trauma Surgeon.**   This is a rather new specialty in medicine. These surgeons generally have four or five years' post-medical-school education, specializing in the care of seriously injured patients.

These groups and individuals are by no means the only health professionals who may be called upon to play a role in the care of a seriously ill or injured person. Before a patient returns to her optimal state of health, numerous other medical specialists and allied health professionals will probably be involved as well.

## DRILLS

There are three ways to learn and maintain Emergency First Care skills: PRACTICE! PRACTICE! PRACTICE! Emergency Medical Professionals complete months, and, in some cases, years of extensive training, but most will admit that their real learning came from internships and clinical rotations where they performed emergency care procedures on actual patients.

Thankfully, First Care Givers generally have few opportunities to perform their skills on actual patients. It is therefore important to hold regular First Care drills. "Somebody's Down Drills" provide a convenient and effective opportunity to enhance the skills and confidence necessary to provide life support when needed.

Such medical drills also allow First Care Givers to continually monitor the effectiveness of their Emergency Medical Response System and to correct deficiencies or problems before an actual emergency takes place.

"Somebody's Down Drills" can be conducted periodically at work and/or at home. There are three components to an effective Medical Response Drill.

## 1. Planning

Drills can be announced (everyone involved knows when it will occur) or they can be unannounced (adding the element of surprise). Regardless of which type, drills need to be properly planned.

Those responsible for arranging a drill can base the drill on previous incidents or "likely to occur" situations. (Try to avoid bizarre or highly hypothetical events.) Individuals selected to be "patients" should be briefed regarding "symptoms and complaints" to be simulated and observers or "evaluators" must be assigned.

## 2. Conduct

When conducting a drill "pseudo victims" and participating responders should try to act as they would in an actual situation. Realism is desirable but great care must be exercised not to actually endanger "victims" or First Care Givers during the drill.

Some risks may sometimes be taken during a real life or death emergency. But actual physical risks are not necessary for effective learning. Nor are they acceptable.

## 3. Evaluation

For a drill to be most beneficial, it must be evaluated.

Every medical drill should be evaluated and constructively critiqued by participants and observers together. Questions to be answered in drill evaluations include:

- Was care appropriate? What could have been done more effectively?
- Were crew communications during the drill effective? What steps should be taken to improve communications?
- Were appropriate medical supplies and equipment available? Were they properly used?

## YOU CAN DO IT!

An adequately developed and properly managed Emergency Medical Response System will provide you with the tools you need to respond to all potential emergency medical situations. Such a system, combined with your ABCS CARE plan, will allow you to support life wherever and whenever needed.

### Don't Let It Happen to You!

Learning and being able to perform Emergency First Care is necessary because people with whom you live and/or work may sustain a sudden illness or injury. But remember, the best way to deal with a medical emergency is to prevent it!

You may not have much control over the health and safety of others, but you certainly can influence your own well-being.

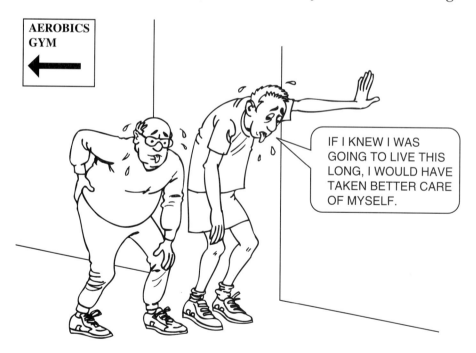

Your plan for medical emergencies is simple: ABCS CARE. Your plan for safe and healthy living (now and through your "golden years") is EESSY:

| | |
|---|---|
| **E**ating | Eat the foods your body needs for energy and vitality. |
| **E**xercise | Do something physical for 15–30 minutes at least three times a week. |
| **S**leep | Get the quality and amount of sleep you need every night. |
| **S**tress management | Condition yourself to cope effectively with the stresses of daily life. Learn to release pent-up stress. |
| **Y**ou | You take care of you. Physically, practice safe behaviors at work, home, and play. Emotionally, make time for fun, family, friends, and, most of all, for you! |

Prevention:

## Don't let it happen to you!

Recognition:

## Check the area!
## Do no harm!
## Make the right call!

Control:

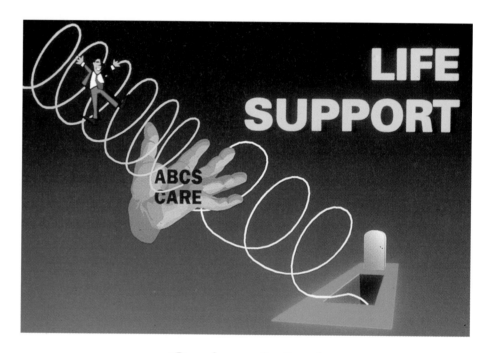

## Be healthy!
## Be safe!
## Be ready!

## You can do it!

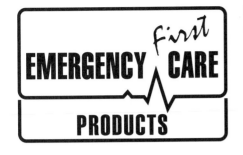

**EMERGENCY** *first* **CARE**
**PRODUCTS**

| TRAINING PRODUCTS | UNIT COST | QTY | TOTAL PRICE |
|---|---|---|---|
| CPR Mini-Manikin | | | |
|    Single Unit (specify male or female) | 39.00 | | |
|    Village (six units) | 222.00 | | |
|    Town (twelve units) | 420.00 | | |
|    City (twenty-four units) | 768.00 | | |
| CPR Baby-Manikin (available December 1995) | Call For Price | | |
| Self Study CPR Video | 29.95 | | |
| **PATIENT CARE PRODUCTS** | | | |
| *Emergency First Care* Deluxe Trauma Kit | 395.00 | | |
| *Emergency First Care* Deluxe Trauma Kit Case ONLY | 99.00 | | |
| *Emergency First Care* Personal Trauma Kit | 69.95 | | |
| CPR MICROKIT™ | 16.95 | | |
| *Emergency First Care*/CPR MICROSHIELD® Personal Protection Pack | 9.95 | | |
| *ChrisKit®* —Emergency Response Kit | 15.95 | | |
| TxO$_2$ Emergency Medical Oxygen Wall Unit | 425.00 | | |
| *Emergency First Care* Poster | 9.95 | | |
| | **SUBTOTAL THIS SIDE** | | |

*For Information on Emergency First Care Instructor Courses
please call Emergency & Safety Programs, Inc. at 1-800-572-2227.*

**Lakeland Medical Products, Co.**
Your Source for Emergency First Care Products

**1 - 8 0 0 - 3 3 6 - 2 5 1 5**

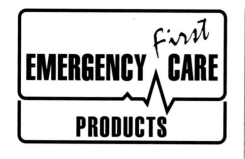

EMERGENCY *First* CARE
PRODUCTS

| PERSONAL USE ITEMS | UNIT COST | QTY | TOTAL PRICE |
|---|---|---|---|
| *Emergency First Care* Pen | 2.00 | | |
| *Emergency First Care* Pen Light | 5.00 | | |
| *Emergency First Care* Lapel Pins | 2.00 | | |
| *Emergency First Care* Patch (3⅞" x 5") | 5.75 | | |
| *Emergency First Care* Decals   4" x 6" | 1.50 | | |
| 2" x 3" | .50 | | |
| *Emergency First Care* Cap | 9.00 | | |
| *Emergency First Care* Shirts<br>(S) (M) (L) (XL) (XXL) | 17.00<br>(plus $2 for XXL) | | |
| *Emergency First Care* Emergency<br>Personal Information Pack | 2.50 | | |
| *Emergency First Care* Check List | 1.50 | | |
| *Emergency First Care* Action Plans | 1.00 | | |

|  |  |
|---|---|
| TOTAL THIS SIDE | |
| TOTAL OTHER SIDE | |
| SUBTOTAL | |
| 5% SHIPPING/HANDLING | |
| Illinois residents add 6.5% sales tax    6.5% ILLINOIS SALES TAX | |
| **TOTAL AMOUNT** | |

## SHIPPING SERVICES

United Parcel Service (UPS) offers 3-Day, 2-Day, and Next Day delivery. Please phone our customer service department for current charges for these special services.

- Please provide recipient's complete street address and phone number with order. UPS does not deliver to PO boxes or APO/FPO addresses. UPS Air Delivery not available for items over 150 pounds.

- Please call 1-800-336-2515 if you need further assistance.

## PAYMENT METHOD

Minimum of $25.00 on all credit card orders

☐ Check          ☐ Money Order          ☐ Visa          ☐ MasterCard

**VISA**          **MasterCard**

Credit Card No.
|  |  |  |  |  |  |  |  |  |  |  |  |  |  |  |  |  |

Card Expiration Date Required

MONTH _____ YEAR _____

Signature

Make checks payable to:  **Lakeland Medical Products, Co.**
P.O. Box 281, Wadsworth, Illinois 60083-0281

# Lakeland Medical Products, Co.
## Your Source for Emergency First Care Products

**1 - 8 0 0 - 3 3 6 - 2 5 1 5**

# EMERGENCY ACTION PLAN

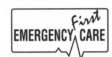

## When Calling for Help...

1. Take a deep breath!
2. Describe the problem.
3. How many victims/patients?
4. Give your name.
5. Give this address and phone number.
6. YOU HANG UP LAST!!!

*You Can Do It!*

EMS _____

POLICE _____

FIRE _____

_____
THIS ADDRESS

_____
THIS PHONE NUMBER

© 1996 Emergency & Safety Programs, Inc., 00 Main Street, Chester, PA 19015 • (610) 872-7447

## Until Help Arrives...
## SUPPORT LIFE

**A** irway
**B** reathing
**C** irculation
**S** pine

**C** ommunicate
**A** void Harm
**R** e-Examine
**E** ncourage

---

### Check The Area
- ☐ Hazards
- ☐ Body Fluids (Latex Gloves?)

### QUIK CHECK™
Look! Listen! Feel!
- ☐ Complaint/Situation
- ☐ Responsive?
- ☐ Body Position

**Airway**
- ☐ Chin Position
- ☐ Obstruction

**Breathing**
- ☐ Look
- ☐ Listen
- ☐ Feel

### Seek Help??
**Circulation**
- ☐ Pulse
- ☐ Bleeding

**Spine**
- ☐ Mechanism of Injury
- ☐ Neck
- ☐ Head
- ☐ Limb Sensation

## LIFE SUPPORT *for* ILLNESS & INJURY

**A** irway
- ☐ Check
- ☐ Open
- ☐ Clear
- ☐ Heimlich
- ☐ Position

**B** reathing
- ☐ Examine
- ☐ Position
- ☐ Fresh Air
- ☐ Crowd Control
- ☐ Oxygen

**C** irculation
- ☐ Pulse
- ☐ Complete Rest
- ☐ Fluid Loss
- ☐ Legs Elevated?
- ☐ Cover

**S** pine
- ☐ Mechanism
- ☐ Survey
- ☐ Don't Move
- ☐ Log Roll??
- ☐ Immobilize

**C** ommunicate
- ☐ Talk to Patient
- ☐ Seek Medical Help
- ☐ Inform Team/Leader
- ☐ Record Care

**A** void Harm
- ☐ No Food/Drink
- ☐ No Medicine (MD?)
- ☐ Be Gentle
- ☐ Secure Body/Parts

**R** e-examine
- ☐ Watch Patient (ABCS)
- ☐ Get the Story
- ☐ Don't Leave Alone
- ☐ Measure Vital Signs

**E** ncourage
- ☐ Emotional Support
- ☐ "Will to Live"
- ☐ Watch What You Say
- ☐ Channel Energies

*You can do it!*

© 1996 Frank J. Poliafico, RN, 00 Main Street, Chester, PA 19015 • (610) 872-7447

### Get the Story
- ☐ What happened?
- ☐ What's wrong/hurts?
- ☐ When did it start?
- ☐ Had this before?
- ☐ Under doctor's care?
- ☐ Take medication?
- ☐ Any allergies?

- ☐ Info from others?
- ☐ Medical I.D.?

### Vital Signs
Conscious
- ☐ Yes   ☐ No

Breathing Rate _____
Pulse Rate _____

*Be Healthy!*
*Be Safe!*
*Be Ready!*

## *for* SUDDEN DEATH

**If Unresponsive:**

- ☐ Yell Out/Send for Help
- ☐ Body Position**???**
- ☐ Open Airway
- ☐ Look, Listen, Feel for Breathing
- ☐ Phone for Help**???**
- ☐ Place Face Shield/Mask**???**
- ☐ Pinch Nostrils**???**
- ☐ Give 2 Slow Breaths
- ☐ Feel for a Pulse
- ☐ Patient on Firm Surface
- ☐ Locate Hand Position
- ☐ Position Your Body
- ☐ 15 Chest Compressions (1$\frac{1}{2}$–2 in.)
- ☐ Give 2 Breaths (see chest rise)
- ☐ Continue 15:2 ratio (5:1 if infant or child)

**Continue CPR until:**

1. Patient's breathing and pulse return.
2. You are relieved by a qualified person.
3. Your own safety is in danger.
4. You are completely exhausted.

### *You can do it!*

## EMERGENCY ACTION PLAN

**IF**

SIGNIFICANT COMPLAINT
MECHANISM OF INJURY
CHANGE IN:
   APPEARANCE
   SPEECH
   CONSCIOUSNESS

**MAKE THE RIGHT CALL**

911
(OR LOCAL
EMERGENCY NUMBER)

**TELL DISPATCHER**

YOUR NAME
THE PROBLEM
HOW MANY PATIENTS
THE LOCATION
THE PHONE NUMBER

*YOU HANG UP LAST!!*

**UNTIL HELP ARRIVES**

*ABCS*
MAKE 'EM THE
**BEST** THEY CAN BE!

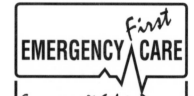

EMERGENCY *first* CARE

*Emergency & Safety Programs*

### *Your Plan*

- ✓ **C**heck **T**he **A**rea
- ✓ Do No Harm
- ✓ Seek Medical Help
- ✓ SUPPORT LIFE